The Long Case OSCE

THE ULTIMATE GUIDE FOR MEDICAL STUDENTS

BETH C WALKER

BSc MBBS PGCMed Ed
Proxime Accessit University of London Gold Medal 2011
Foundation Year 2 Doctor
North Central Thames Foundation School
London

and

MARSHA Y MORGAN

MB ChB FRCP
Principle Research Fellow; Director, Integrated BSc in Clinical Sciences;
Honorary Consultant Physician

U(

B!

Radcliffe Publishing Ltd
St Mark's House
Shepherdess Walk
London N1 7LH
United Kingdom

www.radcliffehealth.com

British Library Cataloguing in Publication Data

A catalogue record for this book is available from the British Library.

ISBN-13: 978 190891 157 5

The paper used for the text pages of this book
is FSC® certified. FSC (The Forest Stewardship
Council®) is an international network to promote
responsible management of the world's forests.

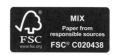

Typeset by Darkriver Design, Auckland, New Zealand
Printed and bound by Hobbs the Printers, Totton, Hants, UK

Contents

CHAPTER 6
Surgical Station   205

Foreword

The clinical examination is sometimes decried as old fashioned and inaccurate, now superseded by imaging and tests. Those who spin this false story have neither honed their skills nor used them to the benefit of their patients, or they would recognise they are wrong. The clinical examination, closely following a detailed, properly focused clinical history, is central to making a diagnosis quickly, or determining the differentials and thereafter directing the use of resources. Understanding the context, set by the patient's story, and then using your eyes, hands, ears and even sense of smell, creates a unique set of observations. Being trained to interpret them, through knowledge of the relationship of symptoms and signs to pathophysiology, is what will make you a doctor. This is why the MBBS long station objective structured clinical examinations (OSCEs) always include systematic examination, and this is also tested in postgraduate examinations by the Royal Colleges. Use this book not only to help you prepare for your examinations but also to guide your learning and practice of these skills, which I have no doubt will remain useful to you throughout your entire professional life.

Professor Jean R McEwan
Professor of Clinical Education
University College London
July 2013

Preface

The long case OSCE examination is, without doubt, one of the most daunting for medical students whenever it is encountered.

Preparing for long case OSCE examinations is not easy and there are few, if any, guides. A solid knowledge base and good clinical skills are clearly needed but do not necessarily guarantee examination success. This can only be ensured if the knowledge and skills are complemented by an ability to interpret the clinical findings, the skill to present them clearly and the confidence to deal with the examiner's questions.

This book is designed as an aid to revision for this examination. Its format is based on a system developed by one of the authors when revising for her own final examinations, a system that was then adopted by several of her friends. In essence, it uses role play with simulated patients to practise clinical examination and presentation skills. The 50 simulated cases presented in this book are representative of those that most often appear in the long case OSCE examination. The questions posed at the end of each of these cases are those most likely to be asked by an examiner, and the answers provided are pitched at the level expected from a student nearing the end of their clinical training.

Suggestions on how to use the book are provided and there is an accompanying video (*see* www.radcliffehealth.com/osce). There is a useful section on how to present clinical findings which makes use of our combined experience of both 'doing it' and of 'observing it done'. Suggested marking schemes are included at the start of each section to provide an idea of what the examiner is expecting to see during the examination process. A clinical 'gem' is included with each case; five handy hints are included at the end of each section and our top 10 tips for OSCE survival are also listed.

This book is not a textbook. It will not provide students with the knowledge they need to pass this examination nor is it intended to replace the experience of examining 'live' patients with senior observation and feedback. However, it will enable students to work either alone or in groups to simulate the examination experience and to hone the skills that need to be honed.

This book should be a valuable resource for medical students in the UK attending universities that use the long case OSCE format. We hope students will enjoy using it and that they will benefit accordingly.

BCW and MYM
July 2013

Acknowledgements

We are extremely grateful to our colleagues who generously reviewed sections of this book:

Mr Ross Davenport

Professor Brian Davidson

Dr Mark Harber

Dr John Hurst

Mr Jay Menon

Dr Richard Orrell

Dr Elysa Speechly-Dick

Dr Richard Stratton.

Any mistakes or inconsistencies are entirely our own.

All men who have turned out worth anything have had the chief hand
in their own education.

Sir Walter Scott (1771–1832)

For
William and Doreen Allison
BCW

Sonia Morgan
MYM

List of Abbreviations

ABPI	ankle brachial pressure index
BP	blood pressure
bpm	beats per minute
CABG	coronary artery bypass graft
CMC	carpometacarpal
CML	chronic myeloid leukaemia
COPD	chronic obstructive pulmonary disease
DIP	distal interphalangeal
FEV$_1$	forced expiratory volume in 1 second
FVC	forced vital capacity
HIV	human immunodeficiency virus
JVP	jugular venous pressure
LUQ	left upper quadrant
MCP	metacarpophalangeal
MRC	Medical Research Council
MTP	metatarsophalangeal
NAFLD	non-alcoholic fatty liver disease
OSCE	objective structured clinical examination
PBC	primary biliary cirrhosis
RIF	right iliac fossa
RUQ	right upper quadrant
SLE	systemic lupus erythematosus
SFJ	saphenofemoral junction
TB	tuberculosis
VSD	ventricular septal defect

About this Book

- There are 50 practice cases in this book divided among the six most commonly examined stations – namely, cardiology, respiratory, abdominal, neurology, musculoskeletal and surgical.

- Each case is intended to typify the sort of patient invited to take part in clinical examinations and, as such, does not necessarily manifest all aspects of a given disease process.

- Every condition has a spectrum of signs and symptoms. However, patients at the very severe end of a disease spectrum are unlikely to be used in examinations unless their condition is stable and they are not unduly distressed by it.

- Each section is preceded by a proposed examination marking scheme that will provide an idea of the aspects of the station the examiner is likely to be asked to mark.

- The significant findings in each case are listed in the order in which they would be encountered if the examination were carried out as per the example marking scheme.

- Important negative findings are also listed for each case. If a clinical finding is not mentioned, you can assume it is normal, e.g. vesicular breath sounds.

- At the end of each case, there are a number of pertinent and commonly asked examination questions centred on the case discussion. Model answers to these are provided at the end of each chapter.

How to Use this Book

The cases presented in this book can be used in a variety of ways:

- To revise typical signs and symptoms of common conditions for the long case OSCEs
- To guide simulation of long station examination technique and the interpretation of findings in a group setting
- To simply exploit the knowledge and experience of people who have survived both taking and examining long case OSCE stations!

If revising in **groups of two**:

- *Student A* will act as the examination candidate and will either actually perform the examination on *Student B* or instead talk through the examination
- *Student B* will act as the patient, will relay the case findings provided to *Student A* at the appropriate time during the examination and will then ask the questions provided.

If revising in **groups of three or more**:

- *Student A* will act as the examination candidate and will either actually perform the examination on *Student B* or instead talk through the examination
- *Student B* will act as the patient
- *Student C* will relay the case findings provided to *Student A* at the appropriate time during the examination and will then ask the questions provided
- Additional students can act as observers and provide feedback.

View the video at www.radcliffehealth.com/osce.

Ten Top Tips for the Long Case OSCE

1. Plan what you are going to wear well ahead of time – make sure you are appropriately dressed, as first impressions count with both patients and examiners. You do not need to look as though you are going to a friend's wedding, but equally you should not look as though you are heading for the beach. Ensure that you are bare below the elbows; piercings, other than earrings, should not be obvious, and midriffs and the tops of underpants should be hidden at all times.

2. Do not forget essential equipment such as your stethoscope and check and check again that you are heading for the right examination centre at the right time on the right day!

3. Make sure you know the time allocation for each OSCE station in advance. Time yourself when practising before the examination to get a good feel for the pace at which you will have to work to complete everything in time. Remember to include the time it will take to introduce yourself to the patients, to provide them with any necessary instructions and to cover them up afterwards.

4. Practise your examination skills over and over again, making sure that you are doing things correctly by asking a doctor to provide feedback.

5. Prepare lists of differential diagnoses for common examination findings when you are revising, e.g. splenomegaly. This will help prevent you being put on the spot when asked for a differential diagnosis when you are already nervous. However, do remember to reorder your list of differentials to best fit the particular patient you are examining – for example, strokes are a much more common cause of facial weakness in an 80-year-old than in a 20-year-old.

6. Similarly, prepare and familiarise yourself with the investigation and management of the conditions most likely to be encountered, e.g. chronic obstructive pulmonary disease (COPD), peripheral neuropathy and thyroid disease.

7. Do not obsess over the diagnosis; the majority of the marks are given for a careful and thorough examination and your ability to identify and interpret the important clinical findings.

8. It is not just the examiner whom you have to impress. Your ability to communicate with the patient is of paramount importance and they will often be asked by the examiner to rate your performance.

9. One or two stations may not go as well as you were hoping. Do not panic if this happens; stay polite and caring towards the patient and carry on with the rest of the examination to the best of your ability. Whatever happens, do not let a 'bad' station affect your overall performance. Put it behind you and start the next station afresh.

10. The OSCEs are designed to allow you to show the examiners that you will make a safe and reliable Foundation Year 1 doctor. That is all the examiners are really interested in. They are certainly not there to deliberately fail you – it involves too much additional paperwork!

Presenting your Findings

The most worrying feature of the long cases is often the thought of presenting your findings at the end of the examination.

Everybody will have different ideas about how they like to present their findings, often based on how they have been taught but also on what has impressed them when they have seen it done by others. The main point is to try to be consistent in what you do, but here are a few other ideas to consider too.

GENERAL TIPS

- Start with an introductory sentence about your patient, stating their age and key comments about their overall condition.

- Be selective about what you include in your presentation – if you start listing every single negative finding the examiner may well 'switch off'.

- If relevant, comment on the patient's functional status as part of your findings.

SYSTEMATIC APPROACH

If you find it easier to present your examination findings in the order you identified them, then you may prefer to use the systematic approach.

The following is an example of this approach:

- *I performed a cardiovascular examination on this 70-year-old gentleman who appeared comfortable at rest with a heart rate of 'X' and blood pressure of 'X'*

- *Around the bedside there was …*

- *On general inspection I found …*

- *On examination of the hands I noted …*

- *On examination of the neck and face there were …*

- *On inspection of the praecordium there was …*

- *On palpation I found …*

- *On auscultation I noted …*

- *On examination of the sacrum and lower limbs for oedema there was …*

- *I did not find any evidence of functional impairment*

- *In summary, this is a 70-year-old gentleman with signs consistent with …*
- *My differential diagnosis is …*

This is a competent and systematic approach which cannot be criticised but is a tad repetitive and sometimes boring to listen to.

'POSITIVE AND NEGATIVE' APPROACH

The 'positive and negative' approach groups your significant positive findings together along with mention of the important negative findings.

The following is an example of this approach:

- *I performed a cardiovascular examination on this 70-year-old gentleman who appeared comfortable at rest*
- *The positive findings of note were …*
- *The negative findings of note were …*
- *I believe this patient's functioning is impaired by his condition because …*
- *In summary, my findings indicate that this patient has …*
- *My differential diagnosis would include …*

This is the thinking man's approach; it is altogether slicker and more professional, provided, of course, that nothing has been missed. Many examiners prefer this method of reporting over others.

'ALL YOUR EGGS IN ONE BASKET' APPROACH

The 'all your eggs in one basket' approach is only suitable if you are as certain as you can be of the diagnosis. You start by stating your diagnosis and then provide the findings to support it.

The following is an example of this approach:

- *I performed a cardiovascular examination on this 70-year-old gentleman who appeared comfortable at rest*
- *I believe he has 'XXX' based on my findings of … and the absence of …*
- *My differential diagnosis would include …*

This is a more robust version of the 'positive and negative' approach and, although impressive, it is an approach that should be used with a considerable degree of caution.

CHAPTER 1

Cardiology Station
Cases 1–9

The secret of getting ahead is getting started.

Mark Twain (1835–1910)

Cardiology Examination
Example Marking Scheme

BEFORE STARTING

- Washes hands
- Introduces self to the patient and states role
- Offers explanation and obtains consent
- Exposes the patient appropriately
- Positions the patient correctly (reclined at 45°)
- Asks whether the patient is in any pain before examining

PERIPHERAL EXAMINATION

- Inspects surroundings for paraphernalia of cardiac disease, e.g. oxygen mask; glyceryl trinitrate spray
- Inspects patient from the end of the bed:
  - ❱ looks for dyspnoea; cyanosis; pallor; malar flush; pulsations in the neck; surgical scars, e.g. midline sternotomy; ankle oedema; obesity and cachexia
- Inspects the hands and arms:
  - ❱ feels for temperature and clamminess; looks for tar staining of the fingers, peripheral cyanosis and clubbing; looks for other signs of infective endocarditis, e.g. Janeway lesions, splinter haemorrhages and Osler's nodes; measures capillary refill time
  - ❱ locates the radial pulse and assesses its rate and rhythm
  - ❱ checks for a slow-rising or collapsing pulse
  - ❱ checks for radio-radial delay and states would check for radio-femoral delay
  - ❱ locates brachial pulse and assesses its character and volume
  - ❱ states intention to measure the blood pressure (BP)
- Inspects the neck and face:
  - ❱ examines the jugular venous pressure (JVP) and measures the height from the sternal angle; states would perform hepatojugular reflex if JVP not visible
  - ❱ locates carotid pulse and assesses its character and volume
  - ❱ inspects the eyes for corneal arcus, xanthelasma and conjunctival pallor; inspects the mouth and tongue for central cyanosis; inspects state of dentition

EXAMINATION OF THE PRAECORDIUM
Inspection

- Inspects the praecordium:
    - ❱ looks for previous scars, visible pacemaker scar and visible apex beat

Palpation

- Locates apex beat, notes any displacement and assesses its quality (normal, tapping, thrusting)
- Palpates for thrills over the aortic and pulmonary areas
- Palpates for heaves over the left parasternal edge
- Palpates for sacral and ankle oedema

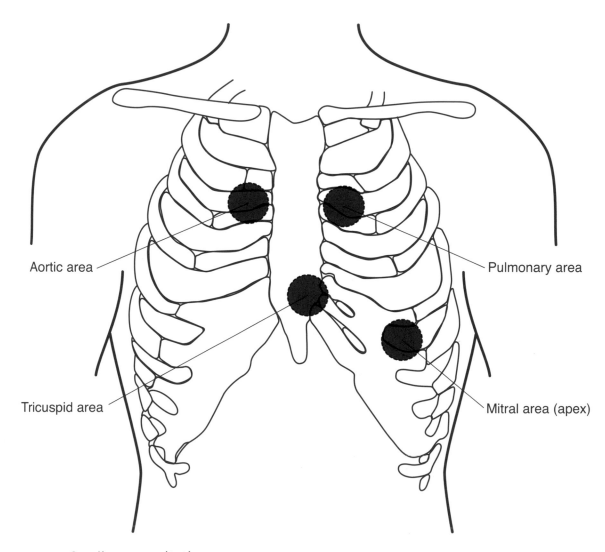

FIGURE 1 Cardiac auscultation areas

Auscultation

- Auscultates the heart sounds over the aortic, pulmonary, tricuspid and mitral areas and times these with the carotid pulse (*see* Figure 1)
- Performs the following manoeuvres:
  - ❭ auscultates over the mitral area for mitral stenosis, using the bell, with the patient in the left lateral position in held expiration
  - ❭ auscultates at the apex using the diaphragm for mitral regurgitation and checks for radiation of the murmur to the axilla
  - ❭ auscultates in the aortic area and at the left sternal edge for aortic regurgitation, using the diaphragm, with the patient leaning forwards in held expiration
  - ❭ auscultates over the aortic area, using the diaphragm, for aortic stenosis; checks for radiation to the carotids
- Auscultates over the carotid arteries for bruits
- Auscultates the lung bases for pulmonary oedema

ADDITIONAL POINTS

- States wish to palpate the peripheral pulses; palpate for an abdominal aortic aneurysm; perform an electrocardiogram; fundoscopy; and dipstick the urine

CONCLUSION

- Thanks the patient and explains that the examination is over
- Offers to help the patient to dress
- Washes hands

DISCUSSION

- Presents findings in a concise and confident manner
- Offers (differential) diagnosis

OVERALL IMPRESSION

- Treats the patient with dignity and respect at all times
- Demonstrates good communication skills
- Performs the examination in a fluent and professional manner

Case 1

Candidate instruction: Please examine this patient's cardiovascular system

Patient information: Mr O, a 66-year-old man

Significant findings on examination:

Inspection: Nothing of note

Peripheral examination: Heart rate regular at 66 beats per minute (bpm)
Slow-rising, low volume pulse
BP 120/85 mmHg

Palpation: Apex beat heaving but not displaced

Auscultation: Ejection systolic murmur, grade 3/6, heard loudest over the aortic area with radiation to the carotids

Important negative findings on examination:

No signs of infective endocarditis
No thrill in the aortic area
No signs of cardiac failure

Present your findings ...

Case 1 Diagnosis:

AORTIC STENOSIS

QUESTION 1

What are the causes of an ejection systolic murmur?

QUESTION 2

What are the causes of aortic stenosis?

QUESTION 3

What symptoms can be associated with aortic stenosis?

In aortic sclerosis, the ejection systolic murmur does not usually radiate to the carotids and the pulse is of normal character and volume

Case 2

Candidate instruction: Please examine this patient's cardiovascular system

Patient information: Mr V, a 63-year-old man

Significant findings on examination:

Inspection:
Midline sternotomy scar
Scar along the distribution of the right long saphenous vein
Audible clicking sound heard from the end of the bed
Bruising of the lower limbs

Peripheral examination:
Heart rate regular at 70 bpm
Pulse of normal character and volume
BP 125/85 mmHg

Palpation:
No abnormalities detected

Auscultation:
S1 metallic and heard loudest in the mitral area
S2 normal

Important negative findings on examination:

No signs of infective endocarditis
Apex beat not displaced and of normal character
No heaves or thrills
No heart murmurs
No signs of cardiac failure

Present your findings ...

Case 2 Diagnosis:

METALLIC MITRAL VALVE REPLACEMENT; CORONARY ARTERY BYPASS GRAFT

QUESTION 1

What are the indications for mitral valve replacement?

QUESTION 2

What are the complications associated with prosthetic valves?

QUESTION 3

What signs of infective endocarditis may be seen on examination?

To help work out which valve has been replaced, time the metallic heart sound with the carotid pulse and note over which area it sounds loudest

Case 3

Candidate instruction: Please examine this patient's cardiovascular system

Patient information: Mrs U, a 77-year-old woman

Significant findings on examination:

Inspection: Midline sternotomy scar

Peripheral examination: Heart rate regular at 74 bpm
Pulse of normal character and volume
BP 124/80 mmHg

Palpation: No abnormalities detected

Auscultation: S1 normal
S2 louder than S1 and of lower pitch
Early diastolic murmur, grade 2/6, heard loudest in the aortic area

Important negative findings on examination:

No signs of infective endocarditis
Apex beat not displaced and of normal character
No heaves or thrills
No signs of cardiac failure

Present your findings ...

Case 3 Diagnosis:

BIOPROSTHETIC AORTIC VALVE REPLACEMENT WITH SIGNS OF VALVULAR DYSFUNCTION (PRESENCE OF AORTIC REGURGITANT MURMUR)

QUESTION 1

What are the indications for aortic valve replacement?

QUESTION 2

What non-invasive investigation could you use to evaluate the direction and velocity of blood flow across the valve?

QUESTION 3

What would be the most important condition to exclude if a patient with a valve replacement developed a new or changing murmur?

In patients with aortic valve replacements, a quiet systolic murmur is likely to be an innocent flow murmur across the prosthesis; an early diastolic murmur is almost always pathological and may be a sign of valve dysfunction

Case 4

Candidate instruction:	Please examine this patient's cardiovascular system; he has a history of shortness of breath on exertion
Patient information:	Mr I, a 68-year-old man

Significant findings on examination:

Inspection:	Nothing of note
Peripheral examination:	Heart rate irregularly irregular at about 80 bpm BP 130/80 mmHg Bilateral pedal pitting oedema
Palpation:	Apex beat thrusting and displaced laterally to the anterior axillary line in the sixth intercostal space
Auscultation:	Pansystolic murmur, grade 3/6, heard loudest at the apex with radiation to the axilla Bibasal lung crepitations

Important negative findings on examination:

No signs of infective endocarditis
JVP not raised
No heaves or thrills
No signs of pulmonary hypertension

Present your findings ...

Case 4 Diagnosis:

MITRAL REGURGITATION WITH ATRIAL FIBRILLATION AND EVIDENCE OF CARDIAC FAILURE (EXERTIONAL DYSPNOEA)

QUESTION 1

What are the causes of a pansystolic murmur?

QUESTION 2

What are the causes of chronic mitral valve regurgitation?

QUESTION 3

What are the causes of acute mitral valve regurgitation?

When auscultating the heart sounds, make sure you time them with a central pulse, e.g. the carotid, and not the radial or brachial

Case 5

Candidate instruction: Please examine this patient's cardiovascular system

Patient information: Mrs C, a 50-year-old woman

Significant findings on examination:

Inspection: Nothing of note

Peripheral examination: Heart rate regular at 76 bpm
Collapsing, large volume pulse
BP 160/68 mmHg

Palpation: Apex beat hyperdynamic and displaced to the anterior axillary line in the sixth intercostal space

Auscultation: Early diastolic murmur, grade 2/6, heard loudest at the lower left sternal edge
Murmur accentuated with patient leaning forwards in held expiration

Important negative findings on examination:

No signs of infective endocarditis
No heaves or thrills
No signs of cardiac failure

Present your findings ...

Case 5 Diagnosis:

AORTIC REGURGITATION

QUESTION 1

What are the causes of a diastolic murmur?

QUESTION 2

What are the causes of aortic regurgitation?

If a patient has aortic regurgitation, look for signs of a possible cause, e.g. infective endocarditis, rheumatoid arthropathy of the hands, the typical spinal deformity of ankylosing spondylitis and skin manifestations of SLE

Case 6

Candidate instruction:	Please examine this patient's cardiovascular system
Patient information:	Mrs D, a 74-year-old woman

Significant findings on examination:

Inspection:	Midline sternotomy scar Scar along the distribution of the left long saphenous vein
Peripheral examination:	Tar staining of the fingers Bilateral corneal arcus Heart rate regular at 70 bpm Pulse of normal character and volume BP 160/85 mmHg
Palpation:	No abnormalities detected
Auscultation:	No abnormalities detected

Important negative findings on examination:

No signs of infective endocarditis
Apex beat not displaced and of normal character
No heaves or thrills
Heart sounds normal with no added sounds or murmurs
No signs of cardiac failure

Present your findings ...

Case 6 Diagnosis:

PREVIOUS CORONARY ARTERY BYPASS GRAFT

QUESTION 1

What cardiac procedures require a midline sternotomy approach?

QUESTION 2

What are the graft harvesting sites for a coronary artery bypass graft (CABG) procedure?

If there is a midline sternotomy scar, make sure you also look for scars in the common graft harvesting sites, e.g. the legs

Case 7

Candidate instruction: Please examine this patient's cardiovascular system

Patient information: Miss B-M, a 26-year-old woman

Significant findings on examination:

Inspection: Nothing of note

Peripheral examination: Heart rate regular at 66 bpm
Pulse of normal character and volume
BP 110/75 mmHg

Palpation: Palpable systolic thrill felt at left lower sternal edge
Left parasternal heave

Auscultation: Pansystolic murmur, grade 4/6, heard at the left
sternal edge radiating to the apex

Important negative findings on examination:

No peripheral or central cyanosis
No signs of infective endocarditis
Apex beat not displaced and of normal character
No signs of cardiac failure
No signs of pulmonary hypertension

Present your findings ...

Case 7 Diagnosis:

VENTRICULAR SEPTAL DEFECT

QUESTION 1

What are the possible complications of an untreated ventricular septal defect (VSD)?

QUESTION 2

What is Eisenmenger's syndrome?

Always think of congenital heart disease when presented with a young cardiology patient – check for clubbing and cyanosis

Case 8

Candidate instruction: Please examine this patient's cardiovascular system

Patient information: Mr R, a 76-year-old man

Significant findings on examination:

Inspection: Bruising of upper and lower limbs

Peripheral examination: Heart rate irregularly irregular at about 70 bpm
BP 170/75 mmHg

Palpation: Difficult to palpate apex beat due to irregular heart rhythm

Auscultation: No abnormalities detected

Important negative findings on examination:

No peripheral or central cyanosis
No signs of infective endocarditis
No signs of cardiac failure
No signs of pulmonary hypertension

Present your findings ...

Case 8 Diagnosis:

ATRIAL FIBRILLATION AND EVIDENCE OF POSSIBLE ANTICOAGULANT THERAPY

QUESTION 1

What assessment score would you use to determine whether a patient with atrial fibrillation should be anticoagulated?

QUESTION 2

What are the complications of atrial fibrillation?

Look for signs of possible causes of atrial fibrillation, e.g. ischaemic heart disease, valvular heart disease and hyperthyroidism

Case 9

Candidate instruction: Please examine this patient's cardiovascular system

Patient information: Mrs F, a 58-year-old woman

Significant findings on examination:

Inspection: Midline sternotomy scar

Peripheral examination: Heart rate regular at 84 bpm
Pulse of normal character and volume
BP 125/80 mmHg

Palpation: No abnormalities detected

Auscultation: S1 normal
S2 metallic heard loudest in the aortic area
Soft systolic murmur, grade 2/6, heard over the aortic area

Important negative findings on examination:

No signs of infective endocarditis
Apex beat not displaced and of normal character
No heaves or thrills
No signs of cardiac failure

Present your findings ...

Case 9 Diagnosis:

METALLIC AORTIC VALVE REPLACEMENT WITH FLOW MURMUR

QUESTION 1

What would be the advantage of using a metallic valve over a bioprosthetic valve?

QUESTION 2

What would be the disadvantage of using a metallic valve over a bioprosthetic valve?

If the metallic heart sound occurs just before the carotid pulsation, this indicates that its origin is the mitral valve whereas if it occurs after the pulsation, this indicates that it is from the aortic valve

5 Handy Hints for the Cardiology Station

1. Avoid making the patient sit backwards and forwards more than once. While the patient is leaning forwards for you to listen for aortic regurgitation, take the opportunity to auscultate the lung bases and check for sacral oedema.

2. If you suspect the patient has had a CABG but you cannot see any evidence of vein harvesting on the legs, then look at the arms to see if there are scars that might indicate use of the *radial arteries* for grafting. If there are no relevant scars on the arms then it is likely that the *left internal mammary* has been used, and this would not leave an external scar.

3. Not all heart procedures require a midline sternotomy approach; check under the left arm for a lateral thoracotomy scar as well. Mitral valve replacements can be done via either approach, as can other procedures.

4. Bioprosthetic valve replacements do not always produce noticeably different heart sound to a native valve. Consider this in your differential in a patient who has scarring consistent with previous cardiac surgery.

5. If you suspect the patient may have had a mitral valve replacement, the location of the apex beat may help provide an idea of the underlying valvular pathology prior to replacement. If the apex beat is displaced laterally, indicating left ventricular dilatation, it is more likely the patient underwent surgery for mitral regurgitation.

Cardiology
Model Answers
Cases 1–9

Case 1

ANSWER 1

The causes of an ejection systolic murmur include:

- Aortic stenosis
- Aortic sclerosis
- Pulmonary stenosis
- Atrial septal defect
- Hypertrophic obstructive cardiomyopathy.

ANSWER 2

The causes of aortic stenosis include:

- Senile calcification (most common)
- Congenital causes (including bicuspid aortic valve, supravalvular stenosis)
- Rheumatic heart disease.

ANSWER 3

The classic triad of symptoms in aortic stenosis is:

- Angina
- Syncope
- Exertional dyspnoea (congestive cardiac failure).

Other symptoms include palpitations, dizziness and fatigue.

Case 2

ANSWER 1

The indications for mitral valve replacement include:

- Mitral regurgitation
- Mitral stenosis
- Mitral valve prolapse (uncommon; surgery indicated only if patient develops severe mitral regurgitation).

ANSWER 2

The complications of prosthetic valves include:

- Structural deterioration, particularly with bioprosthetic valves
- Valve obstruction due to thrombosis formation
- Systemic arterial embolisation
- Infective endocarditis
- Valve-induced haemolysis secondary to turbulent flow
- Increased risk of bleeding if anticoagulated.

ANSWER 3

The signs of infective endocarditis on examination include:

- Fever
- Osler's nodes
- Janeway lesions
- Splinter haemorrhages
- Roth's spots
- Clubbing
- Splenomegaly
- Peripheral arterial emboli, e.g. renal, cerebral, pulmonary
- New-onset heart murmur or change in existing murmur.

Case 3

ANSWER 1

The indications for aortic valve replacement include:

- Aortic stenosis
- Aortic regurgitation.

ANSWER 2

The flow across the heart valves can be assessed using Doppler transthoracic echocardiography.

ANSWER 3

The most important condition to exclude in a patient with a valve replacement who develops a new or changing murmur is infective endocarditis.

Case 4

ANSWER 1

The causes of a pansystolic murmur include:

- Mitral regurgitation
- Tricuspid regurgitation
- VSD.

ANSWER 2

The causes of chronic mitral valve regurgitation include:

- Ischaemic heart disease (secondary to papillary muscle/chordae tendineae dysfunction)
- Functional mitral regurgitation (secondary to any cause of left ventricular dilatation)
- Infective endocarditis
- Rheumatic fever
- Dilated cardiomyopathy
- Mitral valve prolapse
- Connective tissue disorders, e.g. Marfan's syndrome
- Failure of a replacement mitral valve
- Annular calcification (seen in older people).

ANSWER 3

The causes of acute mitral valve regurgitation include:

- Infective endocarditis
- Rupture or dysfunction of papillary muscles/chordae tendineae often secondary to acute myocardial infarction or mitral valve prolapse
- Chest trauma resulting in rupture of the chordae tendineae.

Case 5

ANSWER 1

The causes of an *early* diastolic murmur include:

- Aortic regurgitation
- Pulmonary regurgitation
- Pulmonary regurgitation associated with pulmonary hypertension (Graham Steell murmur).

The causes of a *mid*-diastolic murmur include:

- Mitral stenosis
- Tricuspid stenosis
- Atrial myxoma
- Austin Flint murmur (severe aortic regurgitation).

ANSWER 2

The causes of chronic aortic regurgitation include:

- Idiopathic aortic root dilatation
- Systemic hypertension
- Rheumatic heart disease
- Bicuspid aortic valve
- Infective endocarditis
- Connective tissue disorders, e.g. Marfan's syndrome
- Systemic lupus erythematosus (SLE)
- Seronegative arthritides, e.g. ankylosing spondylitis
- Rheumatoid arthritis
- Drug-induced, e.g. fenfluramine, dopamine agonists
- Syphilitic aortitis.

The causes of acute aortic regurgitation include:

- Infective endocarditis
- Aortic dissection
- Trauma.

Case 6

ANSWER 1

Cardiac procedures requiring a midline sternotomy approach include:

- CABG surgery
- Valve replacement surgery (aortic or mitral)
- Surgical correction of congenital heart defects
- Heart transplant surgery
- Pericardectomy.

ANSWER 2

The harvest sites used for the graft conduit for CABG include:

- Long or short saphenous veins
- Right or left internal mammary (thoracic) arteries
- Radial arteries
- Gastroepiploic artery (rarely).

Case 7

ANSWER 1

The complications of an untreated VSD include:

- Cardiac failure
- Infective endocarditis
- Aortic regurgitation
- Eisenmenger's syndrome.

Small VSDs do not usually require treatment if asymptomatic.

ANSWER 2

Eisenmenger's syndrome arises when a congenital left-to-right shunt, e.g. a VSD, which is not ordinarily associated with cyanosis, results in the development of pulmonary hypertension. This then leads to an increase in the pressure in the right side of the heart causing reversal of the shunt (i.e. from right to left) so that deoxygenated blood bypasses the lungs and causes cyanosis.

Case 8

ANSWER 1

The CHA_2DS_2-VASc score is now used to determine whether patients with atrial fibrillation should be anticoagulated.

C	Congestive heart failure/LV dysfunction	1
H	Hypertension	1
A_2	Age ≥75 years	2
D	Diabetes mellitus	1
S_2	Stroke/TIA/thrombo-embolism	2
V	Vascular disease	1
A	Age 65–74 years	1
Sc	Sex category (female)	1
	Maximum score	9

A score of 2 or more indicates that the patient is in the high-risk stroke category. The European Society of Cardiology guidelines (2010)[1] recommend oral anticoagulant therapy for these patients, unless contraindicated.

ANSWER 2

The complications of atrial fibrillation include:

- Embolic stroke
- Other thromboembolic events
- Heart failure (more likely the atrial fibrillation develops as a result of heart failure than the other way around).

---

1 Camm AJ, Kirchhof P, Lip GY, *et al*. Guidelines for the management of atrial fibrillation: the Task Force for the Management of Atrial Fibrillation of the European Society of Cardiology (ESC). *Europace*. 2010; **12**:1360–420.

Case 9

ANSWER 1

The main advantage of metallic valves is that they are more durable than bioprosthetic valves and so are more commonly used in younger patients.

ANSWER 2

The main disadvantage of metallic valves is that their use requires lifelong anticoagulation therapy.

As a general guide, bioprosthetic valves are recommended for people who cannot or will not take warfarin or who are unlikely to outlive the natural lifespan of the valve; otherwise metallic valves are used.

CHAPTER 2

Respiratory Station
Cases 10–17

All things are difficult before they are easy.

Dr Thomas Fuller (1654–1734)

Respiratory Examination Example Marking Scheme

BEFORE STARTING

- Washes hands
- Introduces self to the patient and states role
- Offers explanation and obtains consent
- Exposes the patient appropriately
- Positions the patient correctly (reclined at 45°)
- Asks whether the patient is in any pain before examining

PERIPHERAL EXAMINATION

- Inspects surroundings for paraphernalia of respiratory disease, e.g. inhalers, nebuliser, sputum pot, oxygen masks, peak flow meters
- Inspects patient from the end of the bed:
  - ❭ looks for respiratory distress, dyspnoea and cyanosis
  - ❭ assesses nutritional status
- Inspects the hands and arms:
  - ❭ feels for temperature; looks for tar staining, clubbing, peripheral cyanosis, tremor
  - ❭ measures radial pulse and assesses rhythm; checks for a bounding pulse
  - ❭ measures respiratory rate
  - ❭ examines for a carbon dioxide retention flap
  - ❭ states intention to measure the BP
- Inspects the neck and face:
  - ❭ examines the JVP
  - ❭ palpates cervical and supraclavicular lymph nodes
  - ❭ inspects the pupils for signs of Horner's syndrome; inspects the tongue for central cyanosis; inspects the conjunctiva for pallor

EXAMINATION OF THE CHEST

Remember to examine both sides of the thorax alternately at the same intercostal level before moving on to the next area, especially during percussion and auscultation.

Inspection

- Inspects the chest:
  - ❯ looks for signs of respiratory distress, e.g. tachypnoea, pursed lips, use of accessory muscles, nasal flaring, intercostal recession
  - ❯ looks for any chest wall scars, deformity or asymmetry
  - ❯ observes chest wall expansion for depth and asymmetry
  - ❯ listens for any audible wheeze or stridor

Palpation

- Palpates position of trachea to check whether central or deviated (warns patient beforehand that this may be uncomfortable)
- Measures crico-sternal distance
- Assesses chest expansion (keeps thumbs off chest wall)
- Palpates for tactile vocal fremitus
- Locates the apex beat checking for displacement
- Palpates for sacral and ankle oedema

Percussion

- Performs percussion of all lung zones including the apices and axillae (*see* Figure 2a and 2b)
- Uses correct technique

Auscultation

- Auscultates breath sounds over all lung zones using diaphragm of stethoscope (*see* Figure 2a and 2b)
- Assesses quality of breath sounds
- Checks for added sounds
- Assesses vocal resonance over all lung zones while patient repeats saying '99'

REPEATS ALL STEPS OF INSPECTION, PALPATION, PERCUSSION AND AUSCULTATION ON THE BACK OF THE CHEST

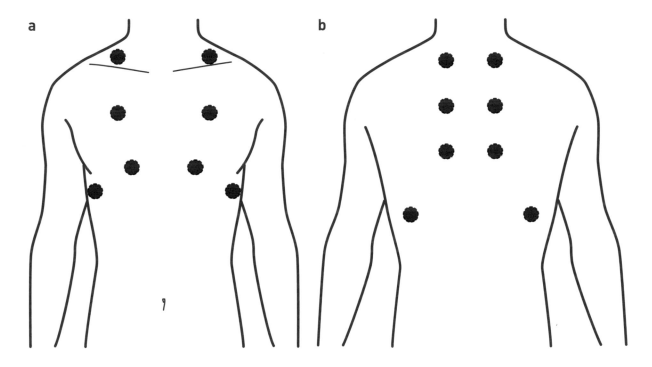

FIGURE 2 Percussion and auscultation areas, front (a) and back (b)

ADDITIONAL POINTS

- States wish to measure oxygen saturation; measure peak flow; and examine the content of any sputum pots

CONCLUSION

- Thanks the patient and explains that the examination is over
- Offers to help the patient to dress
- Washes hands

DISCUSSION

- Presents findings in a concise and confident manner
- Offers (differential) diagnosis

OVERALL IMPRESSION

- Treats the patient with dignity and respect at all times
- Demonstrates good communication skills
- Performs the examination in a fluent and professional manner

Case 10

Candidate instruction:	Please examine this patient's respiratory system; she has a history of progressive shortness of breath on exertion
Patient information:	Mrs C, a 64-year-old woman

Significant findings on examination:

Inspection:	Tachypnoeic at rest Respiratory rate of 22 breaths per minute
Peripheral examination:	Clubbing Peripheral cyanosis Heart rate regular at 70 bpm Pulse of normal character and volume
Palpation:	Chest expansion decreased bilaterally
Percussion:	No abnormalities detected
Auscultation:	Fine late-inspiratory bibasal crepitations

Important negative findings on examination:

No chest wall scars or deformity
No signs of carbon dioxide retention
Trachea central
Apex beat not displaced
Breath sounds vesicular
Vocal resonance normal
No signs of cor pulmonale

Present your findings ...

Case 10 Diagnosis:

PULMONARY FIBROSIS

QUESTION 1

What is the differential diagnosis in this patient?

QUESTION 2

What are the management options for idiopathic pulmonary fibrosis?

QUESTION 3

What would you expect this patient's forced expiratory volume in 1 second/forced vital capacity (FEV_1/FVC) ratio to be?

If you find clubbing and lung crepitations, then you should move idiopathic pulmonary fibrosis and bronchiectasis to the top of your list of differentials

Case 11

Candidate instruction: Please examine this patient's respiratory system; he has a history of progressive shortness of breath on exertion

Patient information: Mr H, a 78-year-old man

Significant findings on examination:

Inspection: Nothing of note

Peripheral examination: Heart rate regular at 88 bpm
Pulse of normal character and volume
Respiratory rate of 18 breaths per minute
JVP raised at 4 cm
Bilateral pitting oedema to the knees

Palpation: Apex beat laterally displaced to the anterior axillary line

Percussion: No abnormalities detected

Auscultation: Fine bibasal crepitations

Important negative findings on examination:

No signs of respiratory distress at rest
No chest wall deformity or scars
No signs of carbon dioxide retention
Trachea central
Normal chest expansion
Breath sounds vesicular
Vocal resonance normal

Present your findings ...

Case 11 Diagnosis:

CONGESTIVE CARDIAC FAILURE

QUESTION 1

What radiographic changes might be seen in left ventricular failure?

QUESTION 2

What system is used to classify the severity of heart failure?

Just because you are asked to perform a respiratory examination does not mean that the findings are necessarily caused by a respiratory condition!

Case 12

Candidate instruction: Please examine this patient's respiratory system

Patient information: Mr N, a 70-year-old man

Significant findings on examination:

Inspection:

Tachypnoeic at rest
Respiratory rate of 22 breaths per minute
Using accessory muscles of respiration and pursing lips
Chest appears hyper-expanded
Reduced crico-sternal distance (<3 fingerbreadths)

Peripheral examination:

Tar staining of the fingers
Heart rate regular at 90 bpm
Pulse of normal character and volume

Palpation:

Reduced chest expansion bilaterally

Percussion:

Percussion note hyper-resonant bilaterally

Auscultation:

Widespread expiratory wheeze

Important negative findings on examination:

No clubbing, cyanosis, chest wall scars or deformity
No signs of carbon dioxide retention
Trachea central
Apex beat not displaced
Breath sounds vesicular
Vocal resonance normal
No signs of cor pulmonale

Present your findings ...

Case 12 Diagnosis:

CHRONIC OBSTRUCTIVE PULMONARY DISEASE

QUESTION 1

What are the management options for COPD?

QUESTION 2

What would you expect this patient's FEV_1/FVC ratio to be?

Remember: COPD does not cause clubbing! If the patient is 'clubbed', respiratory causes include idiopathic pulmonary fibrosis, bronchiectasis, lung abscess and empyema, cystic fibrosis, mesothelioma and lung cancer

Case 13

Candidate instruction: Please examine this patient's respiratory system

Patient information: Mrs O, a 61-year-old woman

Significant findings on examination:

Inspection: Patient wearing a hospital wristband

Peripheral examination:
Tar staining of the fingers
Heart rate regular at 70 bpm
Pulse of normal character and volume
Respiratory rate of 18 breaths per minute

Palpation:
Reduced right basal chest expansion
Decreased tactile vocal fremitus over right base

Percussion: Dullness on percussion of the right lung base

Auscultation:
Diminished breath sounds over right lung base
Decreased vocal resonance over right lung base

Important negative findings on examination:

No signs of respiratory distress at rest
No clubbing, cyanosis, chest wall scars or deformity
No signs of carbon dioxide retention
Trachea central
Apex beat not displaced
No signs of cor pulmonale
Normal examination of left hemithorax

Present your findings ...

Case 13 Diagnosis:

PLEURAL EFFUSION (RIGHT SIDED)

QUESTION 1

How are pleural effusions classified?

QUESTION 2

What are the causes of a pleural effusion?

> Occasionally, stable ward patients are asked to take part in the examinations, so you could see a patient with, for example, a pleural effusion or a resolving pneumonia

Case 14

Candidate instruction: Please examine this patient's respiratory system

Patient information: Mr J, a 70-year-old man

Significant findings on examination:

Inspection: Empty sputum pot by bedside

Peripheral examination: Clubbing
Heart rate regular at 78 bpm
Pulse of normal character and volume
Respiratory rate of 16 breaths per minute

Palpation: No abnormalities detected

Percussion: No abnormalities detected

Auscultation: Bibasal coarse crepitations that alter in character on coughing but do not disappear
Bibasal occasional wheeze

Important negative findings on examination:

No signs of respiratory distress at rest
No cyanosis, chest wall scars or deformity
No signs of carbon dioxide retention
Trachea central
Apex beat not displaced
Normal chest expansion
Normal vocal resonance
No signs of cor pulmonale

Present your findings ...

Case 14 Diagnosis:

BRONCHIECTASIS

QUESTION 1

What are the causes of bronchiectasis?

QUESTION 2

What are the management options for bronchiectasis?

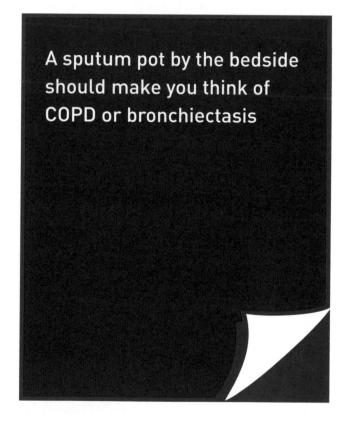

A sputum pot by the bedside should make you think of COPD or bronchiectasis

Case 15

Candidate instruction: Please examine this patient's respiratory system

Patient information: Mr P, a 56-year-old man

Significant findings on examination:

Inspection: Deformity of chest wall – kyphosis and hyperextended neck

Peripheral examination: Heart rate regular at 68 bpm
Pulse of normal character and volume
Respiratory rate of 16 breaths per minute

Palpation: Reduced apical chest expansion

Percussion: No abnormalities detected

Auscultation: Bi-apical fine late-inspiratory crepitations

Important negative findings on examination:

No signs of respiratory distress at rest
No clubbing, cyanosis or chest wall scars
No signs of carbon dioxide retention
Trachea central
Apex beat not displaced
Breath sounds vesicular
Vocal resonance normal
No signs of cor pulmonale

Present your findings ...

Case 15 Diagnosis:

APICAL LUNG FIBROSIS (LIKELY SECONDARY TO ANKYLOSING SPONDYLITIS)

QUESTION 1

What are the causes of apical lung fibrosis?

QUESTION 2

What is the typical radiographic appearance of lung fibrosis?

If there is apical lung fibrosis, look for evidence of possible causes, e.g. signs of ankylosing spondylitis or of old TB, e.g. phrenic nerve crush scars or plombage (NB: these will only be seen in older patients, as these techniques are no longer used)

Case 16

Candidate instruction:	Please examine this patient's respiratory system
Patient information:	Mrs F, a 70-year-old woman

Significant findings on examination:

Inspection:	Faint thoracotomy scar on left thoracic wall Left-sided chest wall deformity underlying scar
Peripheral examination:	Heart rate regular at 75 bpm Pulse of normal character and volume Respiratory rate of 14 breaths per minute
Palpation:	Reduced expansion of the left hemithorax
Percussion:	Dullness to percussion of lower half of left hemithorax
Auscultation:	Diminished breath sounds and decreased vocal resonance over lower half of left hemithorax

Important negative findings on examination:

No signs of respiratory distress at rest
No clubbing or cyanosis
No signs of carbon dioxide retention
Trachea central
Apex beat not displaced
Breath sounds vesicular
No signs of cor pulmonale
Normal examination of right hemithorax

Present your findings ...

Case 16 Diagnosis:

PREVIOUS LEFT LOWER LOBECTOMY

QUESTION 1

Why might this patient have had thoracic surgery?

QUESTION 2

What are the extrapulmonary sites of tuberculosis (TB)?

Make sure you look very carefully for scars on both the anterior and the posterior chest and in the axillae; they can be faint and very easy to miss

Case 17

Candidate instruction:	Please examine this patient's respiratory system
Patient information:	Mr M, a 74-year-old man

Significant findings on examination:

Inspection:	Nasal cannulae and sputum pot at bedside
Peripheral examination:	Tar staining of the fingers Heart rate regular at 90 bpm Pulse of normal character and volume Respiratory rate of 16 breaths per minute JVP raised at 4 cm Blue tinge to the lips and tongue Bilateral pitting oedema to the mid calf Mild sacral oedema
Palpation:	Reduced chest expansion bilaterally Right ventricular heave palpable (left sternal border) Apex beat difficult to feel
Percussion:	No abnormalities detected
Auscultation:	Widespread expiratory wheeze

Important negative findings on examination:

No clubbing, chest wall scars or deformity
No carbon dioxide retention flap
Trachea central
No lung crepitations
Vocal resonance normal

Present your findings ...

Case 17 Diagnosis:

CHRONIC OBSTRUCTIVE PULMONARY DISEASE; SIGNS OF RIGHT HEART FAILURE

QUESTION 1

What is the most likely cause of the right heart failure in this patient?

QUESTION 2

What are the signs of carbon dioxide retention?

The main signs of pulmonary hypertension include a raised JVP with prominent a and v waves, a right ventricular heave and a loud P2

5 Handy Hints for the Respiratory Station

1. Most clinical signs are more easily elicited on examination of the posterior chest. If you are running short of time after the peripheral assessment, examine the back of the chest first to give yourself the best chance of picking up the relevant clinical findings.

2. Remember to ask the patient to breathe through their mouth while you auscultate, rather than though the nose.

3. If you hear crackles on auscultation, ask the patient to cough and then re-auscultate the same area; fine crackles that disappear are most likely caused by airway secretions; coarse crackles that do not disappear but change in nature may be a sign of bronchiectasis.

4. Have a brief look over lung surface anatomy during your revision. It is common for students not to auscultate far enough down the thorax to reach the lung bases and not to auscultate the lateral chest for the right middle lobe.

5. Make sure your findings are consistent with each other, e.g. increased tactile fremitus would not fit with absent breath sounds (*see* Table 1).

TABLE 1 Respiratory Examination Findings Grouped by Disorder

	Pleural effusion	**Pneumothorax**	**Consolidation**
Chest expansion	Reduced	Reduced	Normal or reduced
Tactile fremitus	Reduced or absent	Reduced or absent	Increased
Percussion	Dull (stony)	Hyper-resonant	Dull
Breath sounds	Reduced or absent	Reduced or absent	Bronchial breathing; crepitations
Vocal resonance	Reduced	Reduced	Increased

Respiratory
Model Answers
Cases 10–17

Case 10

ANSWER 1

In the presence of clubbing and fine bibasal crepitations, the most likely diagnosis is idiopathic pulmonary fibrosis; the crepitations heard in bronchiectasis are likely to be coarse.

The causes of bibasal crepitations include:

- Pulmonary oedema
- Pulmonary fibrosis
- Atelectasis
- Pneumonia
- Bronchiectasis.

The causes of basal pulmonary fibrosis include:

- Idiopathic
- Connective tissue disorders, e.g. rheumatoid arthritis, systemic sclerosis
- Drug induced, e.g. methotrexate, amiodarone, bleomycin
- Asbestosis.

ANSWER 2

The mainstay of current treatment is supportive therapy including:

- Pulmonary rehabilitation
- Encouragment smoking cessation
- Oxygen if required
- Early palliative care specialist input.

See National Institute for Health and Clinical Excellence (NICE) guideline CG163 (2013)[2] for further information on current management.

ANSWER 3

The FEV_1/FVC ratio would be normal or increased (>0.7), as pulmonary fibrosis is a restrictive lung disease.

---

2 NICE. Idiopathic pulmonary fibrosis: the diagnosis and management of suspected idiopathic pulmonary fibrosis; NICE guideline 163. London: NICE; 2013. www.nice.org.uk/guidance/CG163

Case 11

ANSWER 1

The radiographic changes that might be seen in left ventricular failure include:

- Upper lobe venous diversion (prominent upper lobe vessels)
- Prominence of hilar pulmonary vasculature
- Interstitial oedema – Kerley B lines
- Alveolar oedema – 'bat wing' appearance
- Cardiomegaly
- Pleural effusions.

The first four are associated more with acute rather than chronic failure.

ANSWER 2

The New York Heart Association Functional Classification[3] is the system used to classify the severity of heart failure based on symptoms.

Class I   Cardiac disease present but causing no limitations on activity. Ordinary physical activity does not cause symptoms.

Class II   Slight limitation of activity. Ordinary physical activity causes symptoms.

Class III Moderate limitation of activity. Less than ordinary physical activity causes symptoms but comfortable at rest.

Class IV   Severe limitation of activity. Symptoms of heart failure present at rest or on minimal exertion.

---

3 Criteria Committee for the New York Heart Association. *Nomenclature and Criteria for Diagnosis of Diseases of the Heart and Great Vessels.* 9th ed. Boston, MA: Little Brown and Company; 1994.

Case 12

ANSWER 1

- The non-pharmacological management for COPD includes:
  - ❱ smoking cessation
  - ❱ pulmonary rehabilitation
  - ❱ long-term oxygen therapy, if patient meets criteria
  - ❱ non-invasive ventilation, if patient meets criteria.
- The pharmacological management for COPD includes:
  - ❱ short- and long-acting inhaled beta-agonists
  - ❱ short- and long-acting inhaled muscarinic antagonists
  - ❱ inhaled corticosteroids
  - ❱ oral theophylline
  - ❱ oral mucolytics
  - ❱ pneumococcal vaccination
  - ❱ annual influenza vaccination
  - ❱ oral steroids, particularly during acute exacerbations
  - ❱ antibiotics if indicated in acute exacerbations.
- The surgical management for COPD can include:
  - ❱ lung volume reduction surgery
  - ❱ bullectomy
  - ❱ lung transplantation.

See NICE guideline CG101 (2010)[4] for current treatment protocols.

ANSWER 2

The patient's FEV_1/FVC ratio would be decreased (<0.7), as COPD is an obstructive lung disease.

---

4 NICE. Chronic obstructive pulmonary disease: management of chronic obstructive pulmonary disease in adults in primary and secondary care (update); NICE guideline 101. London: NICE; 2010. www.nice. org.uk/guidance/CG101

Case 13

ANSWER 1

Pleural effusions are classified as:

- Transudates (<30 g/L protein) and exudates (>30 g/L protein)
- Unilateral or bilateral effusions.

ANSWER 2

The causes of transudative pleural effusions include:

- Cardiac failure
- Cirrhosis
- Nephrotic syndrome
- Malabsorption
- Hypothyroidism
- Peritoneal dialysis.

The causes of exudative pleural effusions include:

- Infection
  - pneumonia
  - pleurisy
  - TB
- Malignancy
  - bronchus/lung
  - pleura
  - metastatic pleural disease
- Pulmonary embolism
- Connective tissue disorders, e.g. rheumatoid arthritis, SLE
- Subphrenic abscess/other subdiaphragmatic pathology, e.g. pancreatitis.

Case 14

ANSWER 1

The commonest cause of bronchiectasis is 'idiopathic'; other causes include:

Congenital:

- Ciliary dysfunction syndromes
  - primary
  - Kartagener's syndrome
  - Young's syndrome
- Cystic fibrosis
- Primary hypogammaglobulinaemia.

Acquired:

- Pneumonia as a complication of, for example, pertussis, measles
- Inhaled foreign body
- Suppurative pneumonias, e.g. klebsiella, *Staphylococcus aureus*
- TB
- Bronchial obstruction, e.g. secondary to lung carcinoma
- Allergic bronchopulmonary aspergillosis
- Chronic aspiration
- Autoimmune diseases, e.g. rheumatoid arthritis, SLE
- Inflammatory bowel disease
- Immunodeficiency, e.g. human immunodeficiency virus (HIV) infection.

ANSWER 2

- The non-pharmacological management includes:
  - chest physiotherapy and postural drainage
  - pulmonary rehabilitation.
- The pharmacological management includes:
  - mucolytics and inhaled bronchodilators
  - antibiotics – for exacerbations and occasionally long-term prophylaxis
  - treatment of underlying condition, e.g. immunoglobulin replacement.

- The surgical management can include resection of localised disease in suitable patients.

See the British Thoracic Society guidelines (2010)[5] for current treatment protocols.

5 Pasteur MC, Bilton D, Hill AT. British Thoracic Society guideline for non-CF bronchiectasis. *Thorax.* 2010; **65** Suppl 1: i1–i58.

Case 15

ANSWER 1

The causes of apical lung fibrosis include:

- TB
- Previous radiotherapy
- Extrinsic allergic alveolitis
- Allergic bronchopulmonary aspergillosis
- Ankylosing spondylitis
- Sarcoidosis
- Silicosis and berylliosis
- Langerhans cell histiocytosis.

ANSWER 2

The classical radiological finding in patients with pulmonary fibrosis is reticulo-nodular shadowing

Case 16

ANSWER 1

The indications for lobectomy include:

- Resection of lung carcinoma
- Mycetoma
- Chronic persistent lung abscess
- Localised lung disease, e.g. bronchiectasis
- TB and its complications
- Trauma.

ANSWER 2

The extrapulmonary sites of TB include:

- Miliary spread
- Gastrointestinal system
- Skeleton, e.g. Pott's disease of the spine
- Central nervous system, e.g. TB meningitis, tuberculoma
- Pericardium
- Genitourinary system, e.g. TB epididymitis
- Lymphatic system, e.g. mycobacterial cervical lymphadenitis
- Skin, e.g. lupus vulgaris.

Case 17

ANSWER 1

In this patient the most likely cause of the right heart failure is cor pulmonale, i.e. right heart failure secondary to pulmonary hypertension caused by chronic lung disease, including COPD, pulmonary emboli and other causes of pulmonary hypertension.

The other causes of right heart failure include:

- Left heart failure
- Mitral stenosis, atrial myxoma
- Other causes of pulmonary hypertension, e.g. pulmonary emboli, primary pulmonary hypertension
- Tricuspid regurgitation
- Congenital heart disease, e.g. tetralogy of Fallot, VSD.

ANSWER 2

The clinical signs of carbon dioxide retention include:

- Bounding character of the pulse
- Flapping tremor
- Altered mental state, e.g. confusion, agitation
- Facial flushing
- Tachypnoea
- Papilloedema.

CHAPTER 3

Abdominal Station
Cases 18–25

Few things are harder to put up with than the annoyance
of a good example.

Mark Twain (1835–1910)

Abdominal Examination Example Marking Scheme

BEFORE STARTING

- Washes hands
- Introduces self to the patient and states role
- Offers explanation and obtains consent
- Exposes the patient appropriately
- Positions the patient correctly (supine with one pillow)
- Asks whether the patient is in any pain before examining

PERIPHERAL EXAMINATION

- Inspects surroundings for paraphernalia of abdominal disease, e.g. vomit bowls, dietary supplements, low-sodium foods/beverages, blood glucose testing kit
- Inspects patient from the end of the bed:
  - ❯ looks for obvious jaundice; stomas; peripheral oedema; nutritional status
- Inspects the hands and arms:
  - ❯ feels for temperature; looks for clubbing, palmar erythema, spider naevi, leukonychia, koilonychia, Dupuytren's contracture; old needle tracks; carpal tunnel release scar; checks for presence of arteriovenous fistulae
  - ❯ examines for the presence of a flapping tremor (asterixis)
- Inspects the neck and face:
  - ❯ examines the JVP with the patient reclined at 45° and measures the height from the sternal angle; states would perform hepatojugular reflex if JVP not visible
  - ❯ looks for telangiectasia, spider naevi, parotid enlargement
  - ❯ examines the eyes for scleral icterus, corneal arcus, conjunctival pallor and xanthelasma; looks for apthous ulcers and macroglossia
  - ❯ smells breath for the foetor of hepatic or renal failure
  - ❯ palpates the left supraclavicular fossa for Virchow's node
  - ❯ looks for parathyroidectomy scar
- Inspects the upper chest:
  - ❯ looks for spider naevi, gynaecomastia; tunnelled dialysis lines

EXAMINATION OF THE ABDOMEN
Inspection

- Inspects the abdomen:
  - ❭ looks for previous scars; stomas; dilated abdominal wall veins; striae; abdominal masses, abdominal distension, obvious abdominal asymmetry; visible peristalsis; hernias; peritoneal dialysis catheter

Palpation

- Asks whether the patient has any pain before starting
- Performs light palpation of the nine segments of the abdomen and observes the patient's face for signs of pain or discomfort
- Performs deep palpation of the nine segments
- Palpates for the presence of hepatomegaly and splenomegaly
- Ballots kidneys
- Palpates for the presence of an abdominal aortic aneurysm
- Palpates for ankle and sacral oedema

Percussion

- Percusses the upper and lower borders of the liver
- Percusses for the presence of splenic dullness
- Percusses over any suspected abdominal masses
- Examines for shifting dullness
- Percusses the suprapubic region if bladder distension is suspected

Auscultation

- Auscultates for bowel sounds
- Auscultates for the presence of renal, hepatic and splenic bruits

ADDITIONAL POINTS

- States wish to examine the hernial orifices and external genitalia; dipstick the urine; and perform a digital rectal examination, if clinically indicated

CONCLUSION

- Thanks the patient and explains that the examination is over
- Offers to help the patient to dress
- Washes hands

DISCUSSION

- Presents findings in a concise and confident manner
- Offers (differential) diagnosis

OVERALL IMPRESSION

- Treats the patient with dignity and respect at all times
- Demonstrates good communication skills
- Performs the examination in a fluent and professional manner

Case 18

Candidate instruction: Please examine this patient's abdomen

Patient information: Mr D, a 55-year-old man

Significant findings on examination:

Inspection:	Mildly jaundiced Moderately malnourished Abdomen moderately distended
Peripheral examination:	Scleral icterus and bilateral palmar erythema Eight spider naevi on chest; bilateral gynaecomastia Prominent and dilated abdominal wall veins Bilateral pitting oedema to mid calf; mild sacral oedema
Palpation:	Mass in left upper quadrant (LUQ) • extends 2 cm below costal margin • moves downwards on inspiration • not possible to feel above it Mass in right upper quadrant (RUQ) and epigastrium • extends 4 cm below costal margin • moves downwards on inspiration • not possible to feel above it
Percussion:	Both masses are dull on percussion Shifting dullness elicited
Auscultation:	No abnormalities detected

Important negative findings on examination:

No abdominal scars
No asterixis or hepatic foetor
No evidence of previous intravenous drug use
No abdominal discomfort/guarding on palpation
Kidneys not palpable
Bowel sounds normal; no abdominal bruits

Present your findings ...

Case 18 Diagnosis:

CHRONIC LIVER DISEASE; SIGNS OF PORTAL HYPERTENSION AND HEPATOCELLULAR DYSFUNCTION

QUESTION 1

What are the causes of chronic liver disease?

QUESTION 2

What are the signs of portal hypertension?

QUESTION 3

Which blood tests could you do to assess the liver's synthetic function?

> In patients with cirrhosis, always check for signs of hepatocellular failure, e.g. jaundice, bruising around venepuncture sites, ascites and hepatic encephalopathy

Case 19

Candidate instruction: Please examine this patient's abdomen

Patient information: Mr F, a 52-year-old man

Significant findings on examination:

Inspection: Faint 15 cm 'hockey stick'-shaped scar in right iliac fossa (RIF)

Peripheral examination: Arteriovenous fistula in left antecubital fossa
- no recent puncture marks

Skin on upper limbs thin and bruised

Palpation: Smooth mass measuring approximately 10 × 6 cm in RIF
- does not move on respiration

Percussion: Mass is dull to percussion

Auscultation: No abnormalities detected

Important negative findings on examination:

No other abdominal scars
JVP not raised
No abdominal discomfort/guarding on palpation
No hepatosplenomegaly
Kidneys not palpable
No ascites
Bowel sounds normal; no abdominal bruits
No peripheral or sacral oedema

Present your findings ...

Case 19 Diagnosis:

RENAL TRANSPLANT; PREVIOUS HAEMODIALYSIS

QUESTION 1

What are the indications for renal transplantation?

QUESTION 2

What complications can patients face following a renal transplant?

> Look for signs of immunosuppressive therapy in transplant patients, e.g. tremor, hirsutism, cushingoid appearance, thin skin and ecchymoses

Case 20

Candidate instruction: Please examine this patient's abdomen

Patient information: Mrs P, a 63-year-old woman

Significant findings on examination:

Inspection: Fullness of the LUQ extending to the midline
Appears pale

Peripheral examination: Conjunctival pallor

Palpation: Smooth mass palpable in LUQ
- extends 10 cm below right costal margin
- moves downwards on inspiration
- not possible to feel above it

Percussion: Mass is dull to percussion

Auscultation: No abnormalities detected

Important negative findings on examination:

No abdominal scars
No excessive bruising
No lymphadenopathy
No abdominal discomfort/guarding on palpation
No hepatomegaly
Kidneys not palpable
No ascites
Bowel sounds normal; no abdominal bruits

Present your findings ...

Case 20 Diagnosis:

MASSIVE SPLENOMEGALY

QUESTION 1

How do you differentiate between an enlarged spleen and a palpable left kidney?

QUESTION 2

What are the causes of massive splenomegaly?

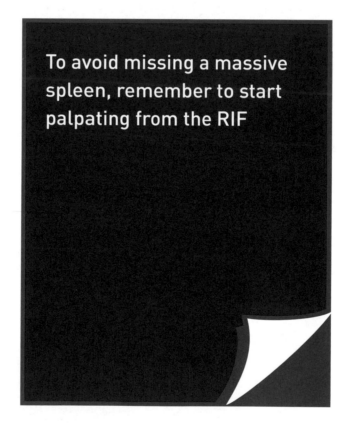

To avoid missing a massive spleen, remember to start palpating from the RIF

Case 21

Candidate instruction: Please examine this patient's abdomen

Patient information: Mr K, a 48-year-old man

Significant findings on examination:

Inspection: Blood glucose testing kit at bedside

Peripheral examination: Several puncture marks in both antecubital fossae
Finger-prick marks

Palpation: Smooth mass palpable in RUQ
- extends 4 cm below costal margin
- moves downwards on inspiration
- not possible to feel above it

Percussion: Mass is dull to percussion

Auscultation: No abnormalities detected

Important negative findings on examination:

Normal body habitus
No abdominal scars
No peripheral stigmata of chronic liver disease
No features of hepatocellular failure
No abdominal discomfort/guarding on palpation
No splenomegaly or other features of portal hypertension
Kidneys not palpable
Bowel sounds normal; no abdominal bruits

Present your findings ...

Case 21 Diagnosis:

MODERATE HEPATOMEGALY AND EVIDENCE OF DIABETES

QUESTION 1

What are the unifying causes of hepatomegaly and diabetes mellitus?

QUESTION 2

Which body systems/organs can be affected in haemochromatosis?

If you suspect haemochromatosis, look for other associated features, e.g. signs of previous venesection, arthropathy, skin pigmentation

Case 22

Candidate instruction:	Please examine this patient's abdomen
Patient information:	Ms P, a 50-year-old woman

Significant findings on examination:

Inspection:	Faint, 20 cm, right-sided scar running obliquely from posterior midline along the lower margin of the ribcage
Peripheral examination:	No abnormalities detected
Palpation:	No abnormalities detected
Percussion:	No abnormalities detected
Auscultation:	No abnormalities detected

Important negative findings on examination:

No other abdominal scars
No abdominal discomfort/guarding on palpation
No abdominal masses
No hepatosplenomegaly
Kidneys not palpable
No ascites
Bowel sounds normal; no abdominal bruits

Present your findings ...

Case 22 Diagnosis:

PREVIOUS RIGHT NEPHRECTOMY

QUESTION 1

What are the indications for a unilateral nephrectomy?

QUESTION 2

What are the main sources of donor organs in the UK?

> Do not panic if you do not find lots of clinical signs; in some patients, there may just be a scar, which will then lead on to a discussion with the examiner

Case 23

Candidate instruction:	Please examine this patient's abdomen
Patient information:	Mr S, an 18-year-old man

Significant findings on examination:

Inspection:	Nothing of note
Peripheral examination:	No abnormalities detected
Palpation:	Smooth mass in the LUQ

- extends 2 cm below costal margin
- moves downwards on inspiration
- not possible to feel above it

Percussion:	Mass is dull to percussion
Auscultation:	No abnormalities detected

Important negative findings on examination:

No peripheral stigmata of chronic liver disease
No abdominal scars
No lymphadenopathy; no pallor
No abdominal discomfort/guarding on palpation
No hepatomegaly
Kidneys not palpable
Bowel sounds normal; no abdominal bruits

Present your findings ...

Case 23 Diagnosis:

MILD SPLENOMEGALY

QUESTION 1

What are the causes of mild splenomegaly?

QUESTION 2

What are the indications for splenectomy?

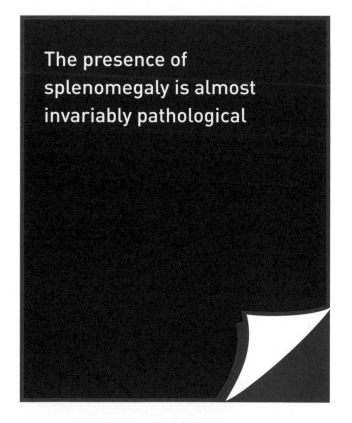

The presence of splenomegaly is almost invariably pathological

Case 24

Candidate instruction:	Please examine this patient's abdomen
Patient information:	Mrs T-J, a 50-year-old woman

Significant findings on examination:

Inspection:	Jaundiced Moderately malnourished
Peripheral examination:	Scleral icterus Skin pigmentation Excoriation marks on arms and trunk Bilateral palmar erythema
Palpation:	Smooth mass palpable in RUQ • extends 4 cm below costal margin • moves downwards on inspiration • not possible to feel above it
Percussion:	Mass is dull to percussion
Auscultation:	No abnormalities detected

Important negative findings on examination:

No abdominal scars

No abdominal discomfort/guarding on palpation

No evidence of hepatocellular failure/portal hypertension

Kidneys not palpable

Bowel sounds normal; no abdominal bruits

Present your findings ...

Case 24 Diagnosis:

HEPATOMEGALY (POSSIBLE PRIMARY BILIARY CIRRHOSIS)

QUESTION 1

What are the indications for liver transplantation?

QUESTION 2

Which blood test is the most specific for primary biliary cirrhosis (PBC)?

In patients with autoimmune liver disease, look for features of other autoimmune disorders, e.g. thyroid disease, Sjögren's syndrome and vitiligo

Case 25

Candidate instruction: Please examine this patient's abdomen

Patient information: Mr L-W, a 42-year-old man

Significant findings on examination:

Inspection: Nothing of note

Peripheral examination: No abnormalities detected

Palpation: Bilateral masses palpable in the flanks
- nodular surface
- ballotable
- non-tender

Percussion: Not easily interpretable

Auscultation: No abnormalities detected

Important negative findings on examination:

No signs of renal replacement therapy
No abdominal scars
No abdominal discomfort/guarding on palpation
No ascites
Bowel sounds normal; no abdominal bruits

NB: it is often difficult to be sure whether the liver and/or spleen are enlarged in these patients

Present your findings ...

Case 25 Diagnosis:

BILATERAL RENAL ENLARGEMENT

QUESTION 1

What are the causes of bilateral renal enlargement?

QUESTION 2

What other clinical features are associated with autosomal dominant polycystic kidney disease?

> Check carefully for scars in the lower abdomen indicating a previous renal transplant – they may be hidden by the patient's clothing

5 Handy Hints for the Abdominal Station

1. Remember to sit the patient forwards to inspect the back and the flanks – otherwise, you may miss signs such as a nephrectomy scar and sacral oedema.

2. If the patient has an arteriovenous fistula, try to determine whether it is functioning. To do this you can look for puncture marks over the fistula, palpate over it for a thrill and auscultate for a bruit.

3. When percussing for the liver, do not forget to percuss the upper border as well. This is vital if you are trying to distinguish between an enlarged liver and a normal liver that has been displaced downwards by hyperinflated lungs.

4. The spleen only becomes palpable in the LUQ when it is approximately three times bigger than normal; if the spleen is not palpable *per abdomen* but is enlarged, there will be dullness to percussion in the ninth intercostal space in the mid-axillary line.

5. As well as the more obvious abdominal scars, look also for smaller, subtler scars left from previous procedures, e.g. paracentesis, peritoneal dialysis, laparoscopy.

Abdominal Model Answers

Cases 18–25

Case 18

QUESTION 1

The causes of chronic liver disease include:

- Alcohol

- Hepatitis B and C infection

- Non-alcoholic fatty liver disease (NAFLD)

- Autoimmune diseases, e.g. autoimmune chronic active hepatitis; PBC; primary sclerosing cholangitis

- Inherited disorders, e.g. haemochromatosis, Wilson's disease

- Drug related, e.g. methotrexate, chlorpromazine.

QUESTION 2

The signs of portal hypertension include:

- Splenomegaly

- Dilated abdominal wall veins and a caput medusae

- Oesophageal varices

- Ascites

- Haemorrhoids.

QUESTION 3

The liver's synthetic function can be assessed by measuring the plasma albumin concentration and the blood prothrombin time/international normalised ratio.

Case 19

QUESTION 1

Renal transplantation is indicated as treatment for end-stage renal failure if the patient is suitable.

The causes of end-stage renal disease (glomerular filtration rate <15 mL/min/ 1.75 m^2) include:

- Diabetic nephropathy
- Glomerulonephritides
- Hypertensive nephropathy
- Polycystic kidney disease.

QUESTION 2

The complications of renal transplantation include:

- Acute or chronic rejection
- Increased risk of atherosclerosis
- Increased risk of infections due to immunosuppressive therapy, e.g. *Cytomegalovirus*, herpes simplex, varicella zoster
- Increased risk of malignancies including skin cancer and lymphoma
- Systemic hypertension
- Side effects of immunosuppressive therapy, e.g. obesity, acne, hirsutism, gout, systemic hypertension, type II diabetes mellitus, adverse lipid profile, nephrotoxicity
- Recurrence of the original pathology in the transplanted organ.

Case 20

QUESTION 1

There are several ways to differentiate the spleen from the left kidney on examination, including:

- The spleen is dull to percussion whereas the kidney is resonant (because of overlying bowel)
- It is not possible to feel above the spleen
- The spleen is not ballotable
- There may be a notch palpable on the anterior margin of the spleen
- The spleen moves inferomedially on inspiration
- The spleen extends towards the RIF when enlarged.

QUESTION 2

The causes of massive splenomegaly (*see* Figure 3) include:

- Chronic myeloid leukaemia (CML)
- Myelofibrosis
- Malaria (rare)
- Gaucher's disease (rare)
- Kala-azar (visceral leishmaniasis – very rare!).

In a patient of this age and sex the most likely differential would be CML.

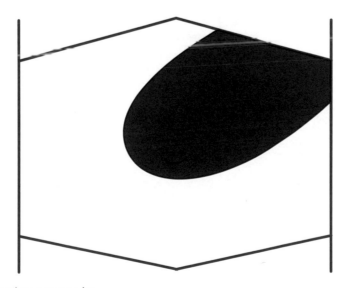

FIGURE 3 Massive splenomegaly

The causes of a moderate splenomegaly (*see* Figure 4) would include the aforementioned causes plus:

- Leukaemias and lymphomas
- Portal hypertension
- Haemolytic anaemias
- Other infections, e.g. Epstein–Barr virus, schistosomiasis
- Storage diseases
- Others, e.g. amyloidosis, sarcoidosis.

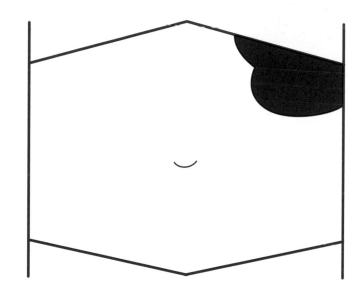

FIGURE 4 Moderate splenomegaly

Case 21

QUESTION 1

The unifying causes of hepatomegaly and diabetes mellitus include:

- NAFLD
- Haemochromatosis.

QUESTION 2

The body systems/organs that can be affected in haemochromatosis include:

- Liver – cirrhosis
- Pancreas – diabetes mellitus and malabsorption
- Heart – cardiomyopathy with or without congestive cardiac failure, arrhythmias
- Joints – arthritis, chondrocalcinosis
- Skin – hyperpigmentation
- Pituitary and testes – hypogonadism and sexual dysfunction.

Case 22

QUESTION 1

The indications for a unilateral nephrectomy in the absence of evidence of chronic renal disease (as in this patient) include:

- Live donation (approximately 1:3 kidney transplants in the UK)
- Renal cell carcinoma
- Renal agenesis/dysgenesis
- Non-functioning kidney, e.g. as a result of renal artery stenosis
- Hydronephrosis
- Pyelonephritis
- Trauma.

QUESTION 2

Sources of organ transplantation are:

- Living related donors
- Donation after brain death
- Non-heart-beating donation after cardiac death
- Living unrelated donors (altruistic or 'daisy chain' donation).

Case 23

QUESTION 1

The causes of mild splenomegaly include:

- Infection, e.g. Epstein–Barr virus, infective endocarditis, brucellosis, malaria
- Lymphoproliferative disorders
- Congenital and acquired haemolytic anaemias, e.g. hereditary spherocytosis, haemoglobinopathies, idiopathic thrombocytopaenic purpura
- Splenic cysts/abscess
- Post-trauma
- Portal hypertension
- Lipid storage disorders
- Amyloidosis
- Sarcoidosis
- Early stages of myeloproliferative disorders, e.g. polycythaemia rubra vera, CML and myelofibrosis.

QUESTION 2

The indications for splenectomy include:

- Traumatic rupture
- Accidental intra-operative rupture
- Severe haemolysis
- Severe thrombocytopaenia
- Severe pancytopaenia
- Splenomegaly causing severe abdominal discomfort/compression of surrounding structures.

Case 24

QUESTION 1

The indications for liver transplantation include:

- Fulminant hepatic failure:
  - ❯ acute viral hepatitis
  - ❯ drug induced, e.g. paracetamol, Ecstasy.
- End-stage cirrhosis:
  - ❯ alcohol
  - ❯ hepatitis B and C infection
  - ❯ NAFLD
  - ❯ autoimmune diseases, e.g. autoimmune chronic active hepatitis, PBC, primary sclerosing cholangitis
  - ❯ inherited disorders, e.g. haemochromatosis, Wilson's disease.
- Primary liver cell cancer fitting specific criteria.

QUESTION 2

The blood test most specific for PBC is the antimitochondrial (M2) antibody.

Case 25

QUESTION 1

The causes of bilateral renal enlargement include:

- Polycystic kidney disease
- Bilateral hydronephrosis
- Lymphoproliferative disorders
- Bilateral renal cell carcinomata (rare)
- Renal amyloidosis
- Tuberous sclerosis (associated with angiomyolipomas and renal cysts)
- Von Hippel–Lindau disease (rare).

QUESTION 2

The other clinical conditions associated with autosomal dominant polycystic kidney disease include:

- Liver cysts
- Pancreatic cysts
- Mitral valve prolapse/Aortic regurgitation
- Intracranial aneurysms
- Diverticular disease.

CHAPTER 4

Neurology Station
Cases 26–34

By failing to prepare, you are preparing to fail.

Benjamin Franklin (1706–1790)

Neurological Examination Upper Limb Example Marking Scheme

When examining the nervous system, it is vital to compare the modality being tested on both sides before continuing to the next component of the examination. This applies to all stages of the neurological examination. Thus, for example, the triceps reflex should be examined on both sides before moving on to examining the biceps reflex.

BEFORE STARTING

- Washes hands
- Introduces self to the patient and states role
- Offers explanation and obtains consent
- Exposes the patient appropriately
- Positions the patient correctly (seated)
- Asks whether the patient is in any pain before examining

INSPECTION

- Inspects bedside surroundings looking for mobility aids and supports, e.g. walking sticks, wheelchair, wrist splints
- Inspects upper limbs:
  - ❱ looks for asymmetry, muscle wasting and fasciculation; scars; skin changes; tremors

TONE

- Assesses tone at shoulder, elbow and wrist
- Tests for supinator catch

POWER

- Tests for pronator drift
- Uses Medical Research Council (MRC) scale[6] (*see* Table 2) to assess the power of:
  - ❱ shoulder abduction and adduction
  - ❱ elbow flexion and extension
  - ❱ wrist flexion and extension

❱ finger flexion, extension, adduction and abduction

❱ thumb abduction, adduction and opposition

❱ power grip and pincer grip strength

TABLE 2 Medical Research Council Scale for Muscle Power[6]

Score	Description
0	No visible muscle contraction
1	Flicker of muscle contraction visible but no movement of joint
2	Movement of muscle at joint when gravity is eliminated
3	Movement of muscle at joint sufficient against effect of gravity
4	Movement overcomes effect of gravity and mild resistance
5	Normal power

REFLEXES

- Elicits triceps, biceps and supinator reflexes using reinforcement if necessary

COORDINATION

- Performs alternate hand test assessing for dysdiadochokinesia
- Performs finger-to-nose test assessing for intention tremor or dysmetria

SENSATION

- Initially demonstrates each method of sensory modality testing on the patient's sternum, asking them to keep their eyes closed
- Demonstrates knowledge of the distribution of dermatomes in the upper limbs (*see* Figure 5):
  ❱ tests pinprick sensation in each dermatome using a neurological pin
  ❱ tests light touch sensation in each dermatome using a monofilament or cotton wool
  ❱ tests proprioception at the distal interphalangeal (DIP) joint of the index

---

6 Medical Research Council. *Aids to the Investigation of the Peripheral Nervous System.* London: Her Majesty's Stationary Office. 1943.

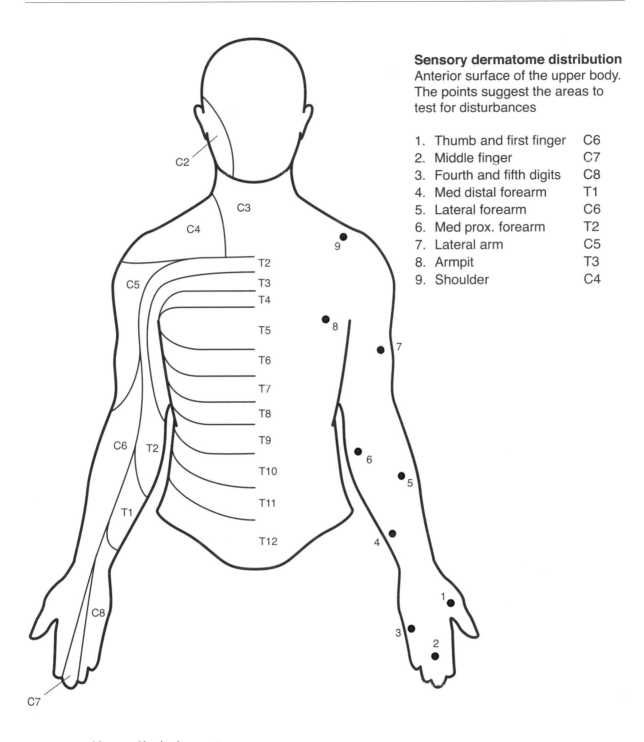

Sensory dermatome distribution
Anterior surface of the upper body.
The points suggest the areas to
test for disturbances

1. Thumb and first finger   C6
2. Middle finger   C7
3. Fourth and fifth digits   C8
4. Med distal forearm   T1
5. Lateral forearm   C6
6. Med prox. forearm   T2
7. Lateral arm   C5
8. Armpit   T3
9. Shoulder   C4

FIGURE 5 Upper limb dermatomes

finger; if proprioception at the DIP joint is impaired, continues to test the next proximal joint until a level is identified

❱ tests vibration sensation using a 128 Hz tuning fork at the DIP joint of the index finger; if vibration sensation at the DIP joint is impaired, continues to test the next proximal joint until a level is identified

❱ states would test temperature sensation using hot and cold test tubes

ADDITIONAL POINTS

- States wish to perform a neurological examination of the lower limbs and cranial nerves

CONCLUSION

- Thanks the patient and explains that the examination is over
- Offers to help the patient to dress
- Washes hands

DISCUSSION

- Presents findings in a concise and confident manner
- Offers (differential) diagnosis

OVERALL IMPRESSION

- Treats the patient with dignity and respect at all times
- Demonstrates good communication skills
- Performs the examination in a fluent and professional manner

---

Useful Hints

- If you find dysdiadochokinesia and an intention tremor, then you should, if you have time, examine for other signs of cerebellar disorder (*see* 'Focused Cerebellar Examination Example Marking Scheme' on p. 125)
- If you find a resting tremor and 'cogwheel' rigidity, then you should, if you have time, perform a focused Parkinson's examination (*see* 'Focused Parkinson's Examination Example Marking Scheme' on p. 127)
- If you do not have time to do these, then make sure you mention to the examiner that this is what you would do to complete your examination

Neurological Examination Lower Limb Example Marking Scheme

When examining the nervous system, it is vital to compare the modality being tested on both sides before continuing to the next component of the examination. This applies to all stages of the neurological examination. Thus, for example, knee extension should be examined on both sides before moving on to exam knee flexion.

BEFORE STARTING

- Washes hands
- Introduces self to the patient and states role
- Offers explanation and obtains consent
- Exposes the patient appropriately
- Positions the patient correctly (standing initially, if possible)
- Asks whether the patient is in any pain before examining

INSPECTION

- Inspects bedside surroundings looking for mobility aids and supports, e.g. foot orthoses, walking sticks, wheelchair
- Inspects lower limbs looking for asymmetry, muscle wasting and fasciculation; scars; skin changes including ulceration; lower limb oedema; presence of a catheter

GAIT

- Assesses gait if the patient is able to walk safely:
  - looks for stride length, smoothness of turning, walking speed and use of any mobility aids
  - assesses nature of gait, e.g. waddling, scissoring, antalgic, circumducting, high stepping
  - examines walking on tiptoes, on heels, and heel-to-toe
- Performs Romberg's test

TONE

- Assesses tone using leg roll and leg lift tests
- Tests for ankle clonus

POWER

- Uses MRC scale[6] (*see* Table 2) to assess the power of:
  - ❯ hip extension, flexion, abduction and adduction
  - ❯ knee extension and flexion
  - ❯ ankle plantarflexion, dorsiflexion, inversion and eversion
  - ❯ big toe extension and flexion

REFLEXES

- Elicits knee and ankle reflexes using reinforcement if necessary
- Elicits plantar responses

COORDINATION

- Asks patient to perform heel-to-shin test

SENSATION

- Initially demonstrates each method of sensory testing on the patient's sternum, asking them to keep their eyes closed
- Demonstrates knowledge of the distribution of dermatomes in the lower limbs (*see* Figure 6):
  - ❯ tests pinprick sensation of each dermatome using a neurological pin
  - ❯ tests light touch sensation of each dermatome using a monofilament or cotton wool
  - ❯ tests proprioception at the DIP joint of the big toe; if proprioception at the DIP joint is impaired, continues to test the next proximal joint until a level is identified
  - ❯ tests vibration sensation using a 128 Hz tuning fork at the DIP joint of the big toe; if vibration sensation at the DIP joint is impaired, continues to test the next proximal joint until a level is identified
  - ❯ states would test temperature sensation using hot and cold test tubes

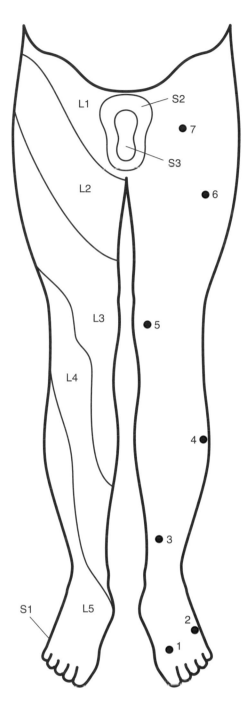

FIGURE 6 Lower limb dermatomes

Sensory dermatome distribution
Anterior surface of the lower body.
The points suggest the areas to
test for disturbances

1.	Big toe – fourth digit	L5
2.	Little toe	S1
3.	Med distal lower leg	L4
4.	Lateral prox. lower leg	L5
5.	Med distal thigh	L3
6.	Lateral prox. thigh	L2
7.	Inner thigh (groin)	L1

ADDITIONAL POINTS

- States wish to perform a neurological examination of the upper limbs and cranial nerves

CONCLUSION

- Thanks the patient and explains that the examination is over
- Offers to help the patient to dress
- Washes hands

DISCUSSION

- Presents findings in a concise and confident manner
- Offers (differential) diagnosis

OVERALL IMPRESSION

- Treats the patient with dignity and respect at all times
- Demonstrates good communication skills
- Performs the examination in a fluent and professional manner

Useful Hints

- If you find impaired coordination or a broad-based gait, then you should, if you have time, examine for other signs of cerebellar disorder (*see* 'Focused Cerebellar Examination Example Marking Scheme' on p. 125)
- If you find a festinant gait, then you should, if you have time, perform a focused Parkinson's examination (*see* 'Focused Parkinson's Examination Example Marking Scheme' on p. 127)
- If you do not have time to do these, then make sure you mention to the examiner that this is what you would do to complete your examination

Cranial Nerve Examination
Example Marking Scheme

When examining the nervous system, it is vital to compare the modality being tested on both sides before continuing to the next component of the examination. This applies to all stages of the neurological examination.

BEFORE STARTING

- Washes hands
- Introduces self to the patient and states role
- Offers explanation and obtains consent
- Exposes the patient appropriately
- Positions the patient correctly (seated)
- Asks whether the patient is in any pain before examining

INSPECTION

- Inspects bedside surroundings looking for walking aids; visual aids; hearing aids
- Inspects patient from the end of the bed:
  - ❭ looks for facial and pupillary asymmetry; abnormal facial movements; abnormal posturing; drooling

CRANIAL NERVE I (OLFACTORY)

- Asks the patient if they have noticed a change in their sense of smell
- States would formally test the olfactory nerve using easily identifiable smell, testing each nostril in turn by occluding the other

CRANIAL NERVE II (OPTIC)

- Asks the patient if they have noticed any changes in their vision in either eye
- Asks the patient if they usually wear glasses or contact lenses, or require use of a white cane or guide dog
- Tests visual acuity in each eye individually using a Snellen chart with patient wearing glasses or contact lenses if used:
  - ❭ if the patient is unable to read the top line of the chart, assesses acuity by testing counting fingers, hand movements and perception of light

- States would test near vision
- States would examine colour vision using Ishihara plates
- Assesses pupillary size, equality and regularity
- Tests pupillary reflexes:
    - ❯ direct, consensual and accommodation
    - ❯ tests for a relative afferent pupillary defect
- Assesses for visual inattention
- Examines temporal and nasal visual fields:
    - ❯ states would map out the blind spot
- States would perform fundoscopy

CRANIAL NERVES III, IV AND VI (OCCULOMOTOR, TROCHLEAR AND ABDUCENS)

- Asks patient if they have double vision or pain on moving their eyes
- Inspects pupillary size, equality and regularity
- Inspects for gaze abnormalities
- Asks the patient to report if they have double vision on examination:
    - ❯ examines all planes of eye movements looking for ophthalmoplegia and nystagmus

CRANIAL NERVE V (TRIGEMINAL)

- Tests light touch sensation across the ophthalmic, maxillary and mandibular branch distributions
- Palpates muscles of mastication while the patient is clenching their teeth
- Tests jaw jerk reflex
- States would test corneal reflex

CRANIAL NERVE VII (FACIAL)

- Inspects for drooping of the mouth or face, asymmetrical forehead wrinkling
- Tests power of the muscles of facial expression
- Asks about any changes in sense of taste
- Asks about any changes in perception of volume of noise

CRANIAL NERVE VIII (VESTIBULOCOCHLEAR)

- Asks the patient about any changes in hearing
- Asks the patient if they use a hearing aid
- Performs a basic test of hearing (whispers a number into one ear while making a distracting noise next to the other ear; asks the patient to recall number heard)
- States would perform Weber's and Rinne's tests using a 512 Hz tuning fork
- States would examine external auditory canals

CRANIAL NERVES IX AND X (GLOSSOPHARYNGEAL AND VAGUS)

- Inspects for symmetry of uvula and soft palate with the patient saying 'aah'
- States would test gag reflex

CRANIAL NERVE XI (SPINAL ACCESSORY)

- Tests power of sternocleidomastoid and trapezius muscles

CRANIAL NERVE XII (HYPOGLOSSAL)

- Inspects tongue while it is at rest in the mouth for fasciculation and wasting
- Inspects for tongue deviation on tongue protrusion
- Asks the patient to move their tongue from side to side

ADDITIONAL POINTS

- States wish to undertake a speech examination and safe swallowing assessment and to perform a neurological examination of the upper and lower limbs

CONCLUSION

- Thanks the patient and explains that the examination is over
- Offers to help the patient to dress
- Washes hands

DISCUSSION

- Presents findings in a concise and confident manner
- Offers (differential) diagnosis

OVERALL IMPRESSION

- Treats the patient with dignity and respect at all times
- Demonstrates good communication skills
- Performs the examination in a fluent and professional manner

Focused Cerebellar Examination Example Marking Scheme

The constellation of signs seen in cerebellar disorders can be remembered using the acronym DANISH:

- **Dysdiadochokinesia**
- **Ataxia**
- **Nystagmus**
- **Intention tremor**
- **Scanning speech**
- **Hypotonia**

There are various ways this examination can be structured; the most important thing is to have a system in place. The example illustrated here is based on a head-to-toe approach.

BEFORE STARTING

- Washes hands
- Introduces self to the patient and states role
- Offers explanation and obtains consent
- Exposes the patient appropriately
- Positions the patient correctly (seated initially)
- Asks whether the patient is in any pain before examining

INSPECTION

- Inspects bedside surroundings looking for walking aids, e.g. walking sticks, wheelchair
- Inspects patient:
  - ❯ looks for nystagmus and truncal ataxia

EYES

- Examines for nystagmus noting the direction of the fast phase
- States would examine for an internuclear ophthalmoplegia

SPEECH

- Examines speech

UPPER LIMBS

- Assesses tone at shoulder, elbow and wrist
- Performs alternate hand testing looking for dysdiadochokinesia
- Performs finger-to-nose test looking for intention tremor and dysmetria
- Examines the upper limbs for the rebound phenomenon
- If paper and pen are available, assesses handwriting for impaired coordination

LOWER LIMBS

- Assesses tone using leg roll and leg lift tests
- Performs the heel-to-shin test

GAIT

- Asks the patient if they are able to walk safely:
  - assesses gait looking for ataxia
  - examines heel-to-toe walking
- States would perform Romberg's test, which will be *negative* in cerebellar ataxia

CONCLUSION

- Thanks the patient and explains that the examination is over
- Offers to help the patient to dress
- Washes hands

DISCUSSION

- Presents findings in a concise and confident manner
- Offers (differential) diagnosis

OVERALL IMPRESSION

- Treats the patient with dignity and respect at all times
- Demonstrates good communication skills
- Performs the examination in a fluent and professional manner

Focused Parkinson's Examination Example Marking Scheme

In a focused examination, the key clinical features of parkinsonism to look for are:

- **Rigidity**
- **Bradykinesia**
- **Resting tremor**
- **Postural instability**

There are various ways this examination can be structured; the most important thing is to have a system in place.

BEFORE STARTING

- Washes hands
- Introduces self to the patient and states role
- Offers explanation and obtains consent
- Exposes the patient appropriately
- Positions the patient correctly (seated initially)
- Asks whether the patient is in any pain before examining

INSPECTION

- Inspects bedside surroundings looking for walking aids, relevant medications
- Inspects patient from the end of the bed:
  - ❯ looks for obvious resting tremor and titubation of the head

GAIT

- Looks for difficulty initiating movement; festinant gait; reduced arm swing; difficulty initiating turning movement; postural instability

FACE

- Inspects for hypomimia (reduced facial expressions); reduced blinking rate; sialorrhoea
- Asks the patient if they have noticed a change in their sense of smell

- Assesses the patient's speech, which tends to be slow, hypophonic and monotonous
- States would perform the Glabellar tap test

UPPER LIMBS

- Inspects for the presence of a resting tremor
  - ❭ observes frequency and nature of resting tremor (typical parkinsonian tremor is described as 4–6 Hz and pill-rolling in nature)
- Assesses tone at the shoulder, elbow and wrist looking for 'lead-pipe' rigidity and 'cogwheeling'
- Examines for bradykinesia:
  - ❭ asks patient to oppose thumb and fingers together repeatedly
  - ❭ looks for slow movement and decreased amplitude of movement on repetition
- If paper and pen are available, assesses handwriting looking for micrographia

LOWER LIMBS

- Inspects for the presence of a resting tremor
- Assesses tone at the knee and ankle looking for lead-pipe rigidity and cogwheeling

CONCLUSION

- Thanks the patient and explains that the examination is over
- Offers to help the patient to dress
- Washes hands

DISCUSSION

- Presents findings in a concise and confident manner
- Offers (differential) diagnosis

OVERALL IMPRESSION

- Treats the patient with dignity and respect at all times
- Demonstrates good communication skills

Case 26

Candidate instruction:	Please examine this patient's upper limb motor neurology
Patient information:	Miss R, a 36-year-old woman

Significant findings on examination:

Inspection:	Nothing of note
Tone:	No abnormalities detected
Power:	No abnormalities detected
Reflexes:	No abnormalities detected
Coordination:	Bilateral intention tremor with past-pointing Bilateral dysdiadochokinesia
If focused cerebellar examination performed:	Ataxic gait Impaired heel-to-toe walking Nystagmus on horizontal gaze bilaterally Speech normal

Important negative findings on examination:

No muscle wasting or fasciculation

Present your findings ...

Case 26 Diagnosis:

BILATERAL CEREBELLAR PATHOLOGY

QUESTION 1

What is the most likely cause of this patient's cerebellar pathology and what other causes could be considered?

QUESTION 2

What are the ophthalmological findings in multiple sclerosis?

> Hypotonia and the presence of pendular reflexes can be signs of cerebellar disease but are subtle and difficult to pick up, especially at undergraduate level

Case 27

Candidate instruction:	Please examine this patient's lower limb motor neurology
Patient information:	Mr B, a 74-year-old man

Significant findings on examination:

Inspection:
Left leg is extended with the left foot held in plantarflexion
Left arm is held in flexion

Gait:
Gait is asymmetrical; slight circumduction of left leg

Tone:
Mild spasticity of left lower limb
Unsustained clonus in left foot

Power:
Reduced power of left lower limb in a pyramidal distribution:
- hip flexion MRC 4/5
- knee flexion MRC 4/5
- ankle dorsiflexion MRC 4/5

Reflexes:
Brisk left knee and ankle reflexes
Upgoing left plantar reflex

Coordination:
Difficult to assess in the left leg because of weakness

Important negative findings on examination:

No muscle wasting or fasciculation
No obvious dysphasia
No facial asymmetry
Normal neurological examination of the right leg

Present your findings ...

Case 27 Diagnosis:

RIGHT UPPER MOTOR NEURON CEREBRAL LESION

QUESTION 1

What is your differential diagnosis in this patient?

QUESTION 2

How would you complete your assessment of this patient's nervous system?

'Clasp-knife' spasticity, as seen in stroke patients, is velocity dependent whereas lead-pipe rigidity, as seen in patients with Parkinson's disease, is velocity independent

Case 28

Candidate instruction: Please examine this patient's lower limb neurology

Patient information: Mr G, a 68-year-old man

Significant findings on examination:

Inspection:	Mild titubation Bilateral resting tremor of hands right > left • approximately 4–6 Hz in frequency • 'pill rolling' in nature
Gait:	Festinant gait, patient takes short and shuffling steps with stooped posture Decreased arm swing and decreased turning speed
Tone:	Bilateral cogwheel rigidity right > left
Power:	No abnormalities detected
Reflexes:	No abnormalities detected
Coordination:	Impaired by bradykinesis
If focused Parkinson's examination performed:	Hypomimia Reduced blink rate Hypophonic speech Bilateral cogwheel rigidity of upper limbs right > left Bradykinesia of upper limbs right > left

Important negative findings on examination:

No asymmetry, muscle wasting or fasciculation
No clonus
No cerebellar signs
No gaze palsies

Present your findings ...

Case 28 Diagnosis:

PARKINSONISM WITH RIGHT-SIDED PREDOMINANCE

QUESTION 1

What are the causes of parkinsonism?

QUESTION 2

What other symptoms might a patient with idiopathic Parkinson's disease display?

If a patient has parkinsonism, you should also test for signs of 'Parkinson's plus' syndromes, e.g. vertical gaze palsy (progressive supranuclear palsy), signs of cerebellar pathology or postural hypotension (multiple-system atrophy)

Case 29

Candidate instruction:	Please examine this patient's upper limb neurology
Patient information:	Mrs J, a 42-year-old woman

Significant findings on examination:

Inspection:	Swollen metocarpophalangeal joints bilaterally Wasting of right thenar eminence
Tone:	No abnormalities detected
Power:	Reduced power of: • right thumb flexion MRC 4/5 • right thumb abduction MRC 4/5 • right thumb opposition MRC 4/5
Reflexes:	No abnormalities detected
Coordination:	No abnormalities detected
Sensation:	Reduced light touch sensation on: • palmar aspect of right thumb, index and middle fingers • lateral palmar aspect of right ring finger
Special tests:	Tinel's test positive on right side Phalen's test positive on right side

Important negative findings on examination:

No scars or muscle fasciculation
Normal neurological examination of the left upper limb

Present your findings ...

Case 29 Diagnosis:

SIGNS OF RIGHT MEDIAN NEUROPATHY (PROBABLE CARPAL TUNNEL SYNDROME)

QUESTION 1

What are the causes of carpal tunnel syndrome?

QUESTION 2

What are the management options for carpal tunnel syndrome?

When looking for previous scars, remember the scar from an open carpal tunnel release procedure is located at the base of the palm of the hand, not on the wrist

Case 30

Candidate instruction: Please examine this patient's cranial nerves

Patient information: Mr A, a 74-year-old man

Significant findings on examination:

Inspection:
Right-sided facial droop
Loss of right-sided facial expression

Cranial nerve VII:
Drooping of the right side of the mouth on smiling
Right-sided weakness in ability to:
- screw up right ocular muscles against resistance
- close right eye
- raise eyebrow against resislance
- blow out right cheek against closed lips

Important negative findings on examination:

No facial scars
No parotid swelling
No abnormalities detected in cranial nerves I–VI, VIII–XII
No alteration in taste sensation or increase in sensitivity to sound

Present your findings ...

Case 30 Diagnosis:

RIGHT-SIDED LOWER MOTOR NEURON FACIAL PALSY

QUESTION 1

How do you differentiate between an upper and lower motor neuron palsy of the facial nerve?

QUESTION 2

What are the causes of a lower motor neuron facial palsy?

QUESTION 3

Why should you ask the patient about their taste and reaction to sound?

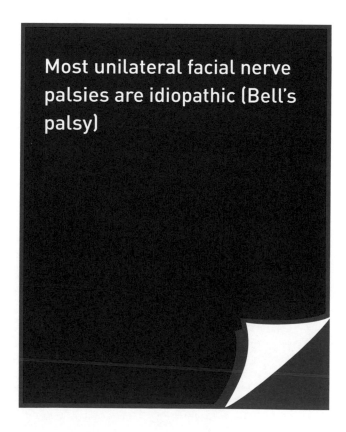

Most unilateral facial nerve palsies are idiopathic (Bell's palsy)

Case 31

Candidate instruction: Please examine this patient's lower limb sensory neurology

Patient information: Mrs P, a 65-year-old woman

Significant findings on examination:

Inspection:
Patient is obese
Blood glucose testing kit at bedside
Healed ulcer scar on left medial malleolus

Pain:
Absent pinprick sensation to the mid calf bilaterally

Light touch:
Loss of light touch sensation to the mid calf bilaterally

Vibration:
Vibration sense absent bilaterally at the first DIP and the metatarsophalangeal (MTP) joints but present at the lateral malleoli

Proprioception:
Proprioception impaired at the first DIP and MTP joints bilaterally but normal at the ankle joints

Important negative findings on examination:

No muscle wasting or joint deformity
If examined, all lower limb pulses palpable bilaterally
If examined, capillary refill time <2 seconds bilaterally

Present your findings ...

Case 31 Diagnosis:

SYMMETRICAL DISTAL SENSORY PERIPHERAL NEUROPATHY

QUESTION 1

What are the causes of peripheral neuropathy?

QUESTION 2

What sensory modality tends to be affected first in diabetic neuropathy?

> If you are running out of time during the sensory examination, testing pain and vibration will cover both the spinothalamic and dorsal column sensory pathways

Case 32

Candidate instruction:	Please examine this patient's lower limb neurology
Patient information:	Mr W, a 32-year-old man

Significant findings on examination:

Inspection:
Foot orthosis by the bedside
Asymmetry of left lower leg musculature
Wasting of anterolateral muscles of left shin (peroneal compartment)

Gait:
Left foot drop
High stepping of the left leg with dragging of the toe

Tone:
No abnormalities detected

Power:
Reduced power of:
- left ankle eversion and dorsiflexion MRC 4/5
- left big toe dorsiflexion MRC 4/5

Reflexes:
No abnormalities detected

Coordination:
No abnormalities detected

Sensation:
Reduced light touch sensation in:
- left anterolateral calf
- dorsum of left foot inclusive of the first web space

Important negative findings on examination:

No scars
No joint deformity or ulcers
Normal neurological examination of the right lower limb
Normal proprioception and vibration bilaterally
If performed, normal hip examination

Present your findings ...

Case 32 Diagnosis:

LEFT COMMON PERONEAL NERVE PALSY

QUESTION 1

What are the causes of a common peroneal nerve palsy?

QUESTION 2

What is the significance of sensory disturbance of the first toe web space?

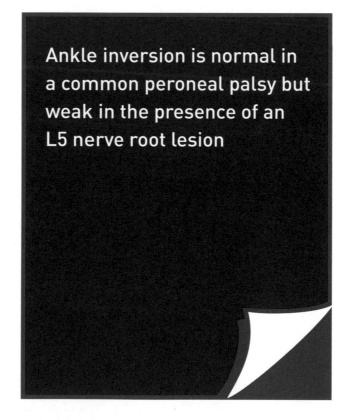

Ankle inversion is normal in a common peroneal palsy but weak in the presence of an L5 nerve root lesion

Case 33

Candidate instruction: Please examine this patient's lower limb motor neurology

Patient information: Mr F, a 50-year-old man

Significant findings on examination:

Inspection:	Zimmer frame at the bedside Bilateral wasting of lower limb musculature
Gait:	Scissoring in nature Patient requires Zimmer frame to mobilise
Tone:	Bilaterally increased tone Bilateral sustained ankle clonus
Power:	Bilaterally reduced power of all movements of the lower limbs MRC 3/5
Reflexes:	Knee and ankle reflexes abnormally brisk bilaterally Bilateral upgoing plantar reflexes
Coordination:	Difficult to assess because of leg weakness

Important negative findings on examination:

No asymmetry, muscle fasciculation or scars
No joint deformity or ulcers
Normal posturing of upper limbs

Present your findings ...

Case 33 Diagnosis:

SPASTIC PARAPLEGIA

QUESTION 1

What are the causes of a spastic paraplegia?

QUESTION 2

How would you complete your examination?

If the patient has sensory or ocular signs, do not list motor neuron disease as a differential – these systems are not affected in this condition

Case 34

Candidate instruction: Please examine this patient's cranial nerves

Patient information: Mrs M, a 38-year-old woman

Significant findings on examination:

Inspection: Nothing of note

Cranial nerve II: Bilateral loss of superior and inferior temporal visual fields

Important negative findings on examination:

No visual inattention
Normal pupillary reflexes
Normal visual acuity
No abnormalities of cranial nerves I, III–XII detected

Present your findings ...

Case 34 Diagnosis:

BITEMPORAL HEMIANOPIA

QUESTION 1

What are the causes of a bitemporal hemianopia?

QUESTION 2

How would you investigate this patient?

> Examine the patient's visual acuity before testing the rest of the optic nerve; trying to examine the visual fields of a patient who is blind may cause distress to the patient and will not gain you any marks!

5 Handy Hints for the Neurology Station

1. The neurology station is often the most feared. Stay calm, be systematic and just present what you find on examination – never try to make up signs to fit in with the clinical picture.

2. Power should be tested using 'like for like' – for example, a patient's finger abduction may appear falsely weak if it is being compared with the strength of the examiner's whole upper limb!

3. Inspection from the end of the bed is key. If you have been asked to examine the lower limbs but the patient also has visible unilateral facial asymmetry, then a possible diagnosis of a cerebrovascular accident should be seriously considered.

4. The hardest thing about the cranial nerve examination can be explaining to the patient what you want them to do without going over time. Try to practise examining the cranial nerves of one of your non-medic friends, as their level of pre-existing knowledge of the examination more closely matches that of a patient.

5. Make sure you know your dermatomes. If you are asked to examine the sensory nervous system, it will soon become obvious if you do not know the correct dermatome distributions. Revise them beforehand and practise.

Neurology Model Answers
Cases 26–34

Case 26

ANSWER 1

The most likely cause of the cerebellar lesion in this young woman is multiple sclerosis.

Other causes that should be considered include:

- Stroke (brainstem)
- Space-occupying lesion
- Alcohol-related cerebellar degeneration
- Drug induced, e.g. phenytoin.

Rarer causes include:

- Non-metastatic neoplastic syndrome (ovary, breast, lung primaries)
- Friedreich's ataxia
- Ataxia telangiectasia
- Spino-cerebellar ataxia.

ANSWER 2

The ophthalmic findings in multiple sclerosis include:

- Resting and/or gaze-evoked nystagmus
- Optic atrophy
- Relative afferent pupillary defect
- Internuclear ophthalmoplegia
- Horizontal and/or vertical gaze palsies.

Case 27

ANSWER 1

The possible causes for the clinical signs seen in this patient include:

- Cerebrovascular accident
- Space-occupying lesion
- Post-traumatic head injury.

ANSWER 2

To complete the assessment of this patient's nervous system, you would need to examine:

- Speech
- Cranial nerves including visual fields and swallow
- Upper limb neurology
- The cardiovascular system, paying particular attention to heart rhythm, BP and carotid artery bruits.

Case 28

ANSWER 1

The causes of parkinsonism include:

- Idiopathic Parkinson's disease
- Lewy body dementia
- Arteriosclerosis ('vascular parkinsonism')
- Drug induced, e.g. haloperidol, chlorpromazine, metoclopramide
- Toxin induced, e.g. manganese, copper (Wilson's disease)
- Multiple-system atrophy
- Post-encephalitic
- Progressive supranuclear palsy
- Corticobasal degeneration
- Dementia pugilistica.

ANSWER 2

The other symptoms that a patient with idiopathic Parkinson's disease might experience include:

- Sialorrhoea
- Anosmia
- Depression
- Visual hallucinations
- Cognitive impairment
- Sleep disturbance
- Dysphagia
- Constipation.

Case 29

ANSWER 1

The causes of carpal tunnel syndrome include:

- Idiopathic
- Pregnancy (and other causes of fluid retention)
- Diabetes mellitus
- Hypothyroidism
- Rheumatoid arthritis and other arthritides of the wrist
- Acromegaly
- Trauma, e.g. previous scaphoid fracture.

ANSWER 2

The management options for carpal tunnel syndrome include:

- Splinting
- Occupational therapy input
- Local corticosteroid injections
- Surgical decompression.

Case 30

ANSWER 1

In upper motor neuron lesions, the forehead is relatively spared because of bilateral innervation of these muscles.

ANSWER 2

The causes of a lower motor neuron facial palsy include:

- Idiopathic (Bell's palsy)
- Chronic middle ear or mastoid infection
- Fracture of the petrous bone
- Parotid tumours
- Lyme disease
- Sarcoidosis
- Leukaemic/Carcinomatous infiltration
- Leprosy
- Acoustic neuroma
- Geniculate herpes (Ramsay Hunt syndrome).

ANSWER 3

The facial nerve gives off both the chordi tympani and stapedial nerves:

- The chorda tympani branch carries taste sensation from the anterior two-thirds of the tongue
- Palsy of the nerve to the stapedius allows wider oscillation of the stapes bone which results in hyperacusis.

Case 31

ANSWER 1

The more common causes of peripheral neuropathy include:

- Idiopathic
- Diabetes mellitus
- Alcohol
- Drug induced, e.g. isoniazid, nitrofurantoin, phenytoin, vincristine and other chemotherapeutic agents
- Chronic renal failure
- Deficiencies of vitamins B_1, B_6 and B_{12}
- Cirrhosis
- Vasculitides, e.g. polyarteritis nodosa
- Connective tissue disorders, e.g. rheumatoid arthritis, SLE.

The less common causes include:

- Hereditary motor and sensory neuropathy (Charcot–Marie–Tooth disease)
- Sarcoidosis
- Amyloidosis
- Porphyria
- Brucellosis
- Paraneoplastic polyneuropathy
- Guillain–Barré syndrome
- Lead poisoning
- Hypothyroidism
- HIV.

ANSWER 2

The first sensory modality affected in diabetic neuropathy tends to be vibration sense.

Case 32

ANSWER 1

Specific causes of common peroneal nerve palsy include:

- Trauma or injury to the knee including during surgery
- Fracture of the fibula
- Compression, e.g. secondary to a tight plaster cast or wearing high knee boots
- Crossing the legs regularly
- Postural pressure on the knee during deep sleep or coma
- Positioning during anaesthesia, especially the lithotomy position.

In addition, consider causes of peripheral mononeuropathy, as described in Case 31, e.g. diabetes mellitus, polyarteritis nodosa, sarcoidosis, hereditary sensory motor neuropathy, leprosy.

ANSWER 2

The significance of sensory disturbance in the first toe web space is that the common peroneal nerve divides into superficial and deep branches. The deep branch supplies sensation to the first web space (between the first and second toes).

Case 33

ANSWER 1

The more common causes of spastic paraplegia include:

- Spinal cord compression
- Vertebral collapse
- Disc prolapse, spondylolisthesis
- Trauma
- Neoplasm (metastases, meningioma, neurofibroma)
- Infection – TB or pyogenic
- Cysts
- Multiple sclerosis
- Motor neuron disease.

Rarer causes include:

- Friedreich's ataxia
- Subacute combined degeneration of the cord
- Syringomyelia
- Anterior spinal artery thrombosis
- Hereditary spastic paraplegia
- HIV.

ANSWER 2

To complete the examination you should:

- Perform a full sensory examination including the perineal area to look for a sensory level
- Test anal tone
- Examine the neurology of the upper limbs and cranial nerves
- Perform a full examination of the spine
- Examine for a palpable bladder.

Case 34

ANSWER 1

The causes of a bitemporal hemianopia include:

- Pituitary tumour
- Craniopharyngioma
- Suprasellar meningioma or cyst
- Anterior communicating artery aneurysm.

Figure 7 illustrates the optic pathways.

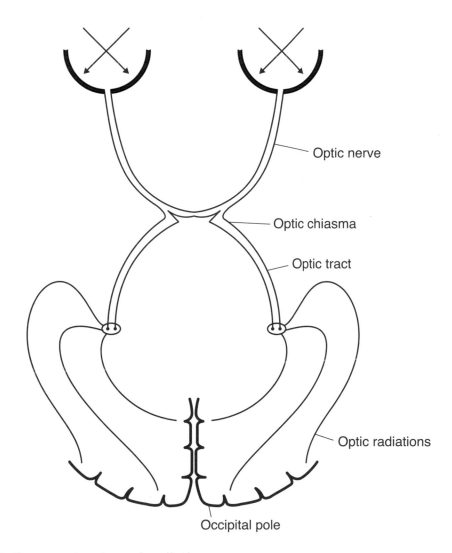

Optic nerve

Optic chiasma

Optic tract

Optic radiations

Occipital pole

FIGURE 7 Optic nerve tracts and radiations

ANSWER 2

The investigation of this patient would include:

- Taking a full history and undertaking a detailed clinical examination
- Blood tests, including prolactin, adrenocorticotropic hormone, growth hormone, thyroid-stimulating hormone, luteinising hormone and follicle-stimulating hormone
- Formal visual-field testing
- Cerebral magnetic resonance imaging with specific views of the suprasellar fossa.

CHAPTER 5

Musculoskeletal Station

Cases 35–42

Far and away the best prize that life offers is the chance to work hard at
work worth doing.

Theodore Roosevelt (1858–1919)

Hand Examination
Example Marking Scheme

Remember that at every stage of the examination you should systematically compare one side with the other.

BEFORE STARTING

- Washes hands
- Introduces self to the patient and states role
- Offers explanation and obtains consent
- Exposes the patient appropriately
- Positions the patient correctly (seated, with hands placed on a pillow, if available)
- Asks whether the patient is in any pain before examining

LOOK

- Inspects the patient's surroundings looking for mobility aids and supports, e.g. hand grabbers, wrist splints
- Inspects the hands
    - ❱ looks for joint swelling and deformity; rheumatoid nodules; gouty tophi; muscle wasting; scars; nail changes including pitting, onycholysis, nail bed infarcts; palmar erythema
- Inspects the elbows
    - ❱ looks and feels for rheumatoid nodules; looks for psoriatic plaques and gouty tophi

FEEL

- Feels the skin temperature over the forearms and hands
- Bimanually palpates interphalangeal, metacarpophalangeal (MCP) and carpal joints for tenderness, bogginess and swelling
- Palpates muscle bulk of the hypothenar and thenar eminences
- Palpates the radial pulses

MOVE

- Assesses active range of movement of wrist flexion and extension
- Tests power of wrist flexion and extension
- Assesses active range of movement of pronation and supination
- Tests power of finger flexion and extension
- Tests power of finger abduction
- States would test power of finger adduction using a piece of paper
- Tests power of thumb abduction and opposition
- Tests power grip and pincer grip strength

SPECIAL TESTS

- Assesses sensation to light touch over relevant areas of skin supplied by the medial, ulnar and radial nerves
- Performs Tinel's test and Phalen's test for carpal tunnel syndrome
- States would perform Froment's test for ulnar nerve paresis
- States would perform Finkelstein's test for De Quervain's tenosynovitis

FUNCTION

- Assesses functional status by asking the patient to, for example, do up a button, pick up a pen, write with a pen

ADDITIONAL POINTS

- States wish to examine the elbow and shoulder joints
- States wish to perform a full neurological examination of the upper limbs

CONCLUSION

- Thanks the patient and explains that the examination is over
- Offers to help the patient to dress
- Washes hands

DISCUSSION

- Presents findings in a concise and confident manner
- Offers (differential) diagnosis

OVERALL IMPRESSION

- Treats the patient with dignity and respect at all times
- Demonstrates good communication skills
- Performs the examination in a fluent and professional manner

Knee Examination
Example Marking Scheme

Remember that at every stage of the examination you should systematically compare one side with the other.

BEFORE STARTING

- Washes hands
- Introduces self to the patient and states role
- Offers explanation and obtains consent
- Exposes the patient appropriately
- Positions the patient correctly (standing initially, if possible)
- Asks whether the patient is in any pain before examining

LOOK

- Inspects bedside surroundings looking for mobility aids and supports, e.g. walking sticks, knee braces
- Inspects patient while standing
  - ❯ looks for asymmetry and muscle wasting; scars; popliteal swellings; valgus or varus deformities
- Assesses gait
  - ❯ looks for stride length, walking speed and use of any mobility aids
  - ❯ looks for evidence of antalgic gait
- Inspects the patient's lower limbs while supine
  - ❯ looks for quadriceps wasting; previous joint replacement or arthroscopy scars; knee joint effusion

FEEL

- Feels the skin temperature over the knee joint
- Palpates the joint lines for tenderness
- Examines for the presence of an effusion
- Palpates the popliteal fossa for a Baker's cyst
- States would measure and compare quadriceps circumference at a fixed point measured from the tibial tuberosity

MOVE

- Assesses active and passive range of movement
- Feels for presence of crepitus while assessing passive movement

SPECIAL TESTS

- Assesses for presence of posterior sag prior to performing drawer tests
- Performs anterior drawer test to assess anterior cruciate ligament
- Performs posterior drawer test to assess posterior cruciate ligament
- Performs valgus stress test to assess medial collateral ligament
- Performs varus stress test to assess lateral collateral ligament
- States would perform McMurray's test

ADDITIONAL POINTS

- States wish to examine the ankle and hip joints
- States wish to perform a full neurovascular examination of the lower limbs

CONCLUSION

- Thanks the patient and explains that the examination is over
- Offers to help the patient to dress
- Washes hands

DISCUSSION

- Presents findings in a concise and confident manner
- Offers (differential) diagnosis

OVERALL IMPRESSION

- Treats the patient with dignity and respect at all times
- Demonstrates good communication skills
- Performs the examination in a fluent and professional manner

Hip Examination Example Marking Scheme

Remember that at every stage of the examination you should systematically compare one side with the other.

BEFORE STARTING

- Washes hands
- Introduces self to the patient and states role
- Offers explanation and obtains consent
- Exposes the patient appropriately
- Positions the patient correctly (standing initially, if possible)
- Asks whether the patient is in any pain before examining

LOOK

- Inspects bedside surroundings looking for mobility aids and special footwear, e.g. walking sticks, built-up shoes
- Inspects patient while standing
  - ❱ looks for asymmetry, quadriceps and gluteal wasting; scars; spinal deformities; alignment of anterior superior iliac spine
- Assesses gait
  - ❱ looks for stride length, walking speed and use of any mobility aids
  - ❱ looks for evidence of antalgic gait, Trendelenburg's gait

FEEL

- Feels the skin temperature over the hip joint
- Palpates over the greater trochanter for tenderness to assess for bursitis

MOVE

- Assesses passive and active range of movement of hip flexion
- Assesses passive range of movement of hip internal and external rotation, adduction and abduction

MEASURE

- Measures apparent leg length from xiphisternum to medial malleolus
- Measures true leg length from anterior superior iliac spine to medial malleolus

SPECIAL TESTS

- Examines for Trendelenburg's sign (*see* Figure 8)
- Performs Thomas test to assess for a fixed flexion deformity (*see* Figure 9)

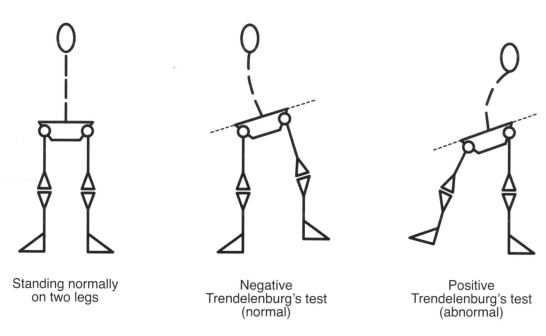

Standing normally on two legs

Negative Trendelenburg's test (normal)

Positive Trendelenburg's test (abnormal)

FIGURE 8 Trendelenburg's sign

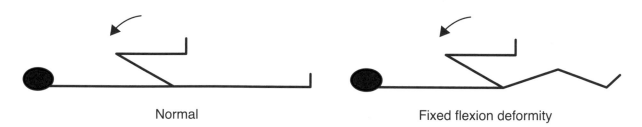

Normal

Fixed flexion deformity

FIGURE 9 Thomas test

ADDITIONAL POINTS

- States wish to examine the knee joints and the spine
- States wish to perform a full neurovascular examination of the lower limbs

CONCLUSION

- Thanks the patient and explains that the examination is over
- Offers to help the patient to dress
- Washes hands

DISCUSSION

- Presents findings in a concise and confident manner
- Offers (differential) diagnosis

OVERALL IMPRESSION

- Treats the patient with dignity and respect at all times
- Demonstrates good communication skills
- Performs the examination in a fluent and professional manner

Spinal Examination
Example Marking Scheme

BEFORE STARTING

- Washes hands
- Introduces self to the patient and states role
- Offers explanation and obtains consent
- Exposes the patient appropriately
- Positions the patient correctly (standing initially, if possible)
- Asks whether the patient is in any pain before examining

LOOK

- Inspects bedside surroundings looking for mobility aids and supports, e.g. Zimmer frame, back brace
- Inspects the patient while standing
  - ❯ looks for spinal asymmetry and deformities; alignment of shoulder and pelvic girdles; muscle wasting; scars
- Assesses gait
  - ❯ looks for stride length, walking speed and use of any mobility aids

FEEL

- Palpates over vertebral processes for tenderness
- Palpates paraspinal musculature for tenderness
- Palpates the sacroiliac joints for tenderness

MOVE

- Assesses active range of movement of cervical extension, flexion, lateral flexion and rotation
- Assesses active range of movement of thoracic rotation and chest expansion
- Assesses active range of movement of lumbar lateral flexion, flexion and extension

SPECIAL TESTS

- Performs Schober's test to assess for reduced range of lumbar movement
- Performs the sciatic nerve stretch test (straight leg raise test) (*see* Figure 10)
- States would perform the femoral nerve stretch test

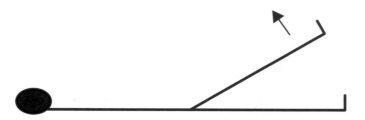

FIGURE 10 Straight leg raise test

ADDITIONAL POINTS

- States wish to examine the hip and shoulder joints
- States wish to perform a full neurovascular examination of the lower limbs

CONCLUSION

- Thanks the patient and explains that the examination is over
- Offers to help the patient to dress
- Washes hands

DISCUSSION

- Presents findings in a concise and confident manner
- Offers (differential) diagnosis

OVERALL IMPRESSION

- Treats the patient with dignity and respect at all times
- Demonstrates good communication skills
- Performs the examination in a fluent and professional manner

Case 35

Candidate instruction:	Please examine this patient's hands
Patient information:	Mrs T, a 50-year-old woman

Significant findings on examination:

Look:	Microstomia
	Perioral telangiectasia
	Bilateral sclerodactyly
	Subcutaneous calcinosis in left fourth and fifth fingertips
Feel:	Skin over fingers feels thickened
Move:	Reduced range of wrist flexion and extension
	Patient unable to fully close fists bilaterally
	Bilaterally reduced grip strength MRC 4/5
Special tests:	No abnormalities detected
Function:	Patient struggles to do up a button

Important negative findings on examination:

No scars, ulceration, muscle wasting, rheumatoid nodules or gouty tophi

No signs of Raynaud's phenomenon

No increased temperature over the joints

No joint tenderness on palpation

Tinel's test and Phalen's test negative

Froment's test negative

Neurovascular system intact

If examined, no crepitations on auscultation of the lungs

Present your findings ...

Case 35 Diagnosis:

LIMITED SYSTEMIC SCLEROSIS (BASED ON THE PATTERN OF SKIN INVOLVEMENT OBSERVED); SIGNS OF FUNCTIONAL IMPAIRMENT

QUESTION 1

What are the clinical features of limited systemic sclerosis?

QUESTION 2

What are the clinical features of diffuse systemic sclerosis?

When you present your findings, avoid using descriptions such as a 'beaky nose', as it can cause distress; say instead that the patient has the characteristic facies of this condition

Case 36

Candidate instruction:	Please undertake a GALS screen and proceed as indicated
Patient information:	Mrs H, a 74-year-old woman

Significant findings on examination:

GALS screening questions:	Reports pain and stiffness in the left hip Does not report any difficulty dressing Reports difficulty with climbing up and down stairs
GALS examination:	Gait – antalgic, requiring use of a walking stick Arms – no abnormalities detected Legs – discomfort on internal rotation of the left hip Spine – no abnormalities detected **Proceed to examine the hips**
Look:	Walking stick at the bedside Antalgic gait; the patient avoids full weight-bearing on the left leg
Feel:	No abnormalities detected
Move:	Reduced range of left hip flexion with discomfort Reduced range of left hip internal rotation with discomfort
Special tests:	No abnormalities detected

Important negative findings on examination:

No scars or muscle wasting
No signs of trochanteric bursitis
No increase in temperature over the joints
No discrepancy in true or apparent leg length
Thomas test negative
Trendelenburg's sign negative
Normal examination of right hip

Present your findings ...

Case 36 Diagnosis:

OSTEOARTHRITIS OF THE LEFT HIP; SIGNS OF FUNCTIONAL IMPAIRMENT

QUESTION 1

What radiographic changes are seen in osteoarthritis?

QUESTION 2

Can you describe how to interpret Trendelenburg's sign?

> When trying to elicit Trendelenburg's sign, make sure you stand close by, as patients, particularly older people, may be very unstable when standing on one leg

Case 37

Candidate instruction: Please examine this patient's knees

Patient information: Mr P-D, a 64-year-old man

Significant findings on examination:

Look: Faint, 8 cm, vertical midline scar on the right knee

Feel: Crepitus palpable over left knee
        Mild effusion in the left knee

Move: Normal range of movement of left knee with mild
        discomfort on flexion
        Mildly reduced range of right knee flexion (115°)

Special tests: No abnormalities detected

Important negative findings on examination:

        Normal gait on inspection
        No walking aids
        No other scars
        No muscle wasting
        No increase in temperature over the joints
        No tenderness on palpation of joint lines
        Cruciate and collateral ligaments intact bilaterally
        If performed, McMurray's test negative

Present your findings ...

Case 37 Diagnosis:

PREVIOUS JOINT REPLACEMENT OF THE RIGHT KNEE; SIGNS OF MILD OSTEOARTHRITIS IN THE LEFT KNEE

QUESTION 1

What questions are important to ask a patient presenting with a knee injury?

QUESTION 2

What is McMurray's test used for?

Remember to palpate the medial and lateral joint lines of the knee separately; it is a common mistake to assess them at the same time, using both hands

Case 38

Candidate instruction:	Please examine this patient's hands
Patient information:	Ms A, a 42-year-old woman

Significant findings on examination:

Look:
Scaly, silvery skin lesions visible along the hairline and on the extensor surfaces of the upper limbs
Bilateral pitting of the fingernails
Swelling of:
- second and third DIP joints of the left hand
- third DIP joint of the right hand

Feel:
Tenderness on palpation of the swollen DIP joints

Move:
Normal grip strength bilaterally; discomfort on gripping tightly with the left hand

Special tests:
No abnormalities detected

Function:
No abnormalities detected

Important negative findings on examination:

No scars, muscle wasting, rheumatoid nodules or gouty tophi
No increase in temperature over the joints
No other joint tenderness
Normal range of movement bilaterally
Tinel's test and Phalen's test negative
Froment's test negative
Neurovascular system intact

Present your findings ...

Case 38 Diagnosis:

PSORIATIC ARTHROPATHY

QUESTION 1

What patterns of joint involvement are seen in patients with psoriatic arthritis?

QUESTION 2

What extra-articular signs can be seen in the hands in patients with psoriatic arthritis?

Remember to look carefully for signs of psoriasis, especially in a patient with nail changes; some patients may only have visible plaques along their hairline

Case 39

Candidate instruction:	Please undertake a GALS screen and proceed as indicated
Patient information:	Mr E, a 65-year-old man

Significant findings on examination:

GALS screening questions:	Reports pain in the right foot Does not report any difficulty with dressing Does not report any difficulty with stairs
GALS examination:	Gait – mildly antalgic, no walking aids used Arms – no abnormalities detected Legs – swelling of first MTP joint of right foot; discomfort on squeezing right MTP joints Spine – no abnormalities detected **Proceed to examine the feet**
Look:	Mildly antalgic gait Two tophi on the medial aspect of the right hallux Right first MTP joint swollen and laterally deviated
Feel:	Tenderness on palpation of right first MTP joint
Move:	Range of dorsiflexion and plantarflexion of right hallux limited by discomfort

Important negative findings on examination:

No scars, muscle wasting or rheumatoid nodules
No other tophi
No increase in temperature or erythema of skin over the joints
Normal examination of left foot
Neurovascular system intact

Present your findings ...

Case 39 Diagnosis:

GOUTY ARTHRITIS (CHRONIC)

QUESTION 1

What are the causes of a red, acutely inflamed joint?

QUESTION 2

What would be your first-line investigation if considering a diagnosis of septic arthritis?

QUESTION 3

What would you find on examination of the synovial fluid in an acute attack of gout?

If you suspect gout, make sure to look carefully for tophi; sites include the hands, feet, olecranon bursae, Achilles tendons and the ear helices

Case 40

Candidate instruction:	Please examine this patient's hands
Patient information:	Miss K, a 72-year-old woman

Significant findings on examination:

Look:	Bilateral swellings at the base of both thumbs over the first carpometacarpal (CMC) joints
	Bony swellings over the right second and fifth DIP joints and the left second DIP joint consistent with Heberden's nodes
	Bilateral wasting of the dorsal interossei muscles
Feel:	Discomfort on palpation of the first CMC joints bilaterally
Move:	Reduced range of wrist flexion and extension bilaterally
	Bilaterally reduced grip strength MRC 4/5
Special tests:	No abnormalities detected
Function:	No abnormalities detected

Important negative findings on examination:

No scars, rheumatoid nodules or gouty tophi

No increase in temperature or erythema of skin over the joints

No other joint swellings or deformities

Tinel's test and Phalen's test negative

Froment's test negative

Neurovascular system intact

Present your findings ...

Case 40 Diagnosis:

OSTEOARTHRITIS OF THE HANDS

QUESTION 1

What signs of osteoarthritis can be seen in the hands?

QUESTION 2

What are the management options for osteoarthritis?

When examining the wrists and hands, make sure you are constantly looking at the patient's face to check for any signs of pain or discomfort

Case 41

Candidate instruction:	Please undertake a GALS screen and proceed as indicated
Patient information:	Mr G, a 50-year-old man

Significant findings on examination:

GALS screening questions:	Reports stiffness of the spine Does not report any difficulty with dressing Does not report any difficulty with stairs
GALS examination:	Gait – no abnormalities detected Arms – no abnormalities detected Legs – no abnormalities detected Spine – kyphosis and loss of lumbar lordosis, reduced range of lumbar flexion **Proceed to examine the spine**
Look:	Kyphosis and loss of lumbar lordosis
Feel:	Discomfort on palpation of sacroiliac joints
Move:	Significantly reduced range across all planes of movement of cervical, thoracic and lumbar spine
Special tests:	Schober's test positive (increase of 4 cm on measuring lumbar flexion)

Important negative findings on examination:

No scars, muscle wasting, rheumatoid nodules or gouty tophi
No scoliosis
No vertebral or paraspinal muscle tenderness
Sciatic and femoral nerve stretch tests negative
If examined, no crepitations on auscultation of lungs

Present your findings ...

Case 41 Diagnosis:

ANKYLOSING SPONDYLITIS

QUESTION 1

What are the management options for patients with ankylosing spondylitis?

QUESTION 2

What are the extra-spinal complications of ankylosing spondylitis?

If you have time, look for extra-spinal complications of ankylosing spondylitis, e.g. auscultate for signs of lung fibrosis and aortic regurgitation, palpate the Achilles tendons for tenderness and swelling

Case 42

Candidate instruction:	Please examine this patient's hands
Patient information:	Ms M, a 56-year-old woman

Significant findings on examination:

Look:	Bilateral swollen MCP joints
	Bilateral ulnar deviation of the fingers
	Bilateral 'swan neck' deformities of the second and third fingers
	Bilateral wasting of the dorsal interossei muscles
	Several rheumatoid nodules over both olecranon processes
Feel:	Tender MCP joints bilaterally with increase in temperature and erythema of the overlying skin
Move:	Significantly reduced range of wrist flexion and extension
	Reduced power of:
	● thumb abduction MRC 4/5
	● finger extension, flexion and abduction MRC 4/5
	● grip and pincer strength MRC 4/5
Special tests:	No abnormalities detected
Function:	Patient is unable to do up buttons

Important negative findings on examination:

No scars, gouty tophi or nail changes
No swelling or tenderness of interphalangeal joints
Tinel's test and Phalen's test negative
Froment's test negative
Neurovascular system intact

Present your findings ...

Case 42 Diagnosis:

RHEUMATOID ARTHRITIS OF THE HANDS; SIGNS OF FUNCTIONAL IMPAIRMENT

QUESTION 1

What are the management options for patients with rheumatoid arthritis?

QUESTION 2

What radiographic changes are seen in rheumatoid arthritis?

QUESTION 3

What are the extra-articular manifestations of rheumatoid arthritis?

One of the most important things to comment on when presenting your findings in a patient with arthritis is their functional status

5 Handy Hints for the Musculoskeletal Station

1. If asked to perform a GALS screen, do not forget to ask the three screening questions in addition to undertaking the examination.

2. It is very important to expose the patient adequately when performing the GALS screen and joint examinations. Always check that the patient is comfortable undressing to their underwear before you start; remember, the patients who attend finals will know what to expect.

3. You may find that you have not been provided with any equipment with which to assess hand function, e.g. a pen, and the patient may not be wearing anything buttoned. If so, you can improvise and assess function by making one of your hands into a fist and asking the patient to grip it and try to turn it as if it were a doorknob.

4. If you suspect the patient has rheumatoid arthritis, look for signs of the possible side effects of medications, e.g. thinning of the skin and/or increased bruising from corticosteroids or mouth ulcers from methotrexate.

5. Perform the posterior sag test before doing the drawer tests when examining the knee ligaments. If the posterior sag test is positive, this can indicate a posterior cruciate ligament rupture. When the posterior cruciate ligament is ruptured, the anterior drawer test will be falsely positive.

Musculoskeletal
Model Answers
Cases 35–42

Case 35

ANSWER 1

The clinical features of limited systemic sclerosis include:

- Raynaud's phenomenon
- Skin thickening limited to the face, lower arms (below elbows) and lower legs (below knees)
- Arthropathy
- Some patients may present with a constellation of features that used to be referred to by the acronym CREST:
  - ❱ Calcinosis
  - ❱ Raynaud's phenomenon
  - ❱ Esophageal dysmotility
  - ❱ Sclerodactyly
  - ❱ Telangiectasia
- The limited form of the disease typically has a slower and less severe disease course than the diffuse form
- Some patients may develop complications more often associated with the diffuse form of the disease – namely, pulmonary hypertension and interstitial lung disease
- Limited systemic sclerosis may occasionally be associated with hypothyroidism and PBC.

ANSWER 2

The clinical features of diffuse systemic sclerosis include:

- Raynaud's phenomenon
- Widespread cutaneous involvement
- Arthropathy
- Interstitial lung disease; pulmonary hypertension
- Myocardial fibrosis; pericardial effusion
- Oesophageal dysmotility, gastroparesis, reflux oesophagitis
- Small bowel involvement leading to malabsorption
- Renal crises (accelerated hypertension leading to acute kidney injury)
- Chronic vasculopathy leading to chronic renal failure.

Case 36

ANSWER 1

The radiographic changes seen in osteoarthritis include:

- Loss of joint space
- Subarticular sclerosis
- Osteophyte formation
- Subchondral cysts.

ANSWER 2

A positive Trendelenburg's sign indicates weak hip abductors. The patient is asked to stand up and to weight bear on their affected leg by lifting their unaffected leg. If a patient with weak left hip abductors lifts their right leg while standing on their affected left leg, the pelvis will sag to the right.

Case 37

ANSWER 1

The questions that are important to ask a patient presenting with a knee injury include:

- How did you injure your knee?
- Do you have pain in your knee?
- If you have pain in your knee, where is it most painful?
- What makes the pain worse?
- Have you noticed any swelling of your knee?
- Has your knee ever felt unstable or given way?
- Does your knee ever lock (i.e. get stuck in one position)?
- Have you injured your knee previously?

ANSWER 2

McMurray's test is used to assess for the presence of meniscal tears.

Case 38

ANSWER 1

There are five different presenting patterns of joint involvement in psoriatic arthritis:

- Rheumatoid-like polyarthropathy
- Distal interphalangeal joint arthropathy
- Asymmetrical oligoarthropathy
- Spondyloarthropathy plus or minus sacroiliitis
- Psoriatic arthritis mutilans.

ANSWER 2

Extra-articular signs in the hand in patients with psoriatic arthritis include:

- Nail pitting
- Nail discolouration and thickening
- Onycholysis (lifting of the nail off the nail bed)
- Visible psoriatic plaques
- Dactylitis.

Case 39

ANSWER 1

The most important differential to exclude in a patient with a red, acutely inflamed joint would be septic arthritis. Other causes include:

- Crystal arthropathies (gout and pseudogout)
- Reactive arthritis
- Haemarthrosis
- Trauma
- Monoarthritic presentation of rheumatoid arthritis.

ANSWER 2

The first-line investigation of a possible septic arthritis would be joint aspiration and examination of the synovial fluid, including Gram stain and culture.

ANSWER 3

The synovial fluid during an acute attack of gout contains negatively birefringent needle-shaped crystals.

Case 40

ANSWER 1

The clinical signs of osteoarthritis in the hands include:

- Heberden's nodes (DIP joints)
- Bouchard's nodes (proximal interphalangeal joints)
- Muscle wasting of the hands
- Subluxation of first CMC joint resulting in squaring of the thumbs.

ANSWER 2

The management options for osteoarthritis include:

- General measures:
  - ❭ weight loss
  - ❭ ensuring access to appropriate information and understanding of the condition
  - ❭ exercise and physiotherapy
  - ❭ walking aids
  - ❭ appropriate footwear
  - ❭ heat- or cool-pack therapy
  - ❭ transcutaneous electrical nerve stimulation.
- Medical treatment:
  - ❭ paracetamol as first-line oral analgesia
  - ❭ topical non-steroidal anti-inflammatory drugs
  - ❭ continuation up the pain ladder if needed
  - ❭ topical capsaicin
  - ❭ intra-articular steroid injections if pain moderate to severe.
- Surgical treatment:
  - ❭ joint replacement surgery.

See NICE guideline CG59 (2008)[7] for further information on management options.

---

7 NICE: The care and management of osteoarthritis in adults: NICE guideline 59. London: NICE; 2008. www.nice.org.uk/guidance/CG59

Case 41

ANSWER 1

- The general management options for ankylosing spondylitis include:
  - ❯ regular exercise
  - ❯ physiotherapy.
- The medical management options include:
  - ❯ analgesia (non-steroidal anti-inflammatory drugs unless contraindicated)
  - ❯ tumour necrosis factor alpha inhibitors (under the care of a rheumatologist).
- Spinal surgery is not routinely indicated as a treatment option.

ANSWER 2

The extra-spinal complications of ankylosing spondylitis include:

- Apical lung fibrosis
- Anterior uveitis
- Sacroiliitis
- Achilles tendonitis
- Arthritis (seronegative, usually mono- or oligo-arthritis of large joints)
- Cardiac arrhythmias, e.g. atrioventricular nodal block
- Aortic regurgitation.

Case 42

ANSWER 1

- The general management options for rheumatoid arthritis include:
  - ❯ physiotherapy
  - ❯ occupational therapy, home adaptations and dexterity aids
  - ❯ splints.
- The medical management is usually directed by a rheumatologist and depends on disease activity; options include:
  - ❯ analgesia
  - ❯ corticosteroids
  - ❯ disease-modifying anti-rheumatic drugs
  - ❯ biological agents, e.g. infliximab (tumour necrosis factor alpha inhibitor); rituximab (anti-CD20 monoclonal antibody); tocilizumab (anti-interleukin 6).
- Surgical management may be indicated in certain situations, e.g.
  - ❯ carpal tunnel release
  - ❯ joint replacement.

ANSWER 2

The radiographic changes seen in rheumatoid arthritis include:

- Narrowing of joint spaces
- Juxta-articular osteopaenia
- Bony erosions
- Soft-tissue swelling
- Joint subluxation.

ANSWER 3

The extra-articular manifestations of rheumatoid arthritis include:

- Rheumatoid nodules (subcutaneous and pulmonary)
- Pulmonary fibrosis and obliterative bronchiolitis
- Pleural and pericardial effusions
- Accelerated atherosclerosis
- Peripheral neuropathy, especially carpal tunnel syndrome
- Conjunctival sicca, episcleritis and scleritis
- Vasculitis
- Anaemia
- Amyloidosis.

CHAPTER 6

Surgical Station

Cases 43–50

Nothing is really work unless you would rather be doing something else.

JM Barrie (1860–1937)

Surgical Abdominal Examination Example Marking Scheme

BEFORE STARTING

- Washes hands
- Introduces self to the patient and states role
- Offers explanation and obtains consent
- Exposes the patient appropriately
- Positions the patient correctly (supine with one pillow)
- Asks whether the patient is in any pain before examining

PERIPHERAL EXAMINATION

- Inspects surroundings for paraphernalia of abdominal disease, e.g. vomit bowl; dietary supplements
- Inspects patient from the end of the bed
  - ❯ looks for obvious jaundice; stomas; nutritional status
- Inspects the hands and arms
  - ❯ feels for temperature; looks for clubbing, palmar erythema, Dupuytren's contracture, leukonychia and koilonychia; spider naevi; checks for presence of arteriovenous fistulae
- Inspects the neck and face
  - ❯ looks for telangiectasia, spider naevi, parotid enlargement
  - ❯ examines the eyes for scleral icterus, corneal arcus, conjunctival pallor and xanthelasma; looks for apthous ulcers and macroglossia
  - ❯ palpates the left supraclavicular fossa for Virchow's node
- Inspects the chest
  - ❯ looks for spider naevi and gynaecomastia

EXAMINATION OF THE ABDOMEN
Inspection

- Inspects the abdomen
  - ❯ looks for previous scars; stomas; dilated abdominal wall veins; striae; abdominal asymmetry, abdominal masses, abdominal distension; visible peristalsis; hernias
  - ❯ asks the patient to cough, looking for presence of abdominal hernias

Palpation

- Asks whether the patient has any pain before starting
- Performs light palpation of the nine segments of the abdomen and observes the patient's face for signs of pain or discomfort
- Performs deep palpation of the nine segments
- Palpates for the presence of hepatomegaly and splenomegaly
- Ballots kidneys
- Palpates for the presence of an abdominal aortic aneurysm
- States would examine hernial orifices and external genitalia

Percussion

- Percusses the upper and lower borders of the liver
- Percusses for the presence of splenic dullness
- Percusses over any suspected abdominal masses
- Examines for shifting dullness
- Percusses suprapubic region if bladder distension is suspected

Auscultation

- Auscultates for bowel sounds
- Auscultates for the presence of hepatic, renal and splenic bruits

ADDITIONAL POINTS

- States would like to perform a digital rectal examination, if clinically indicated, and dipstick the urine

CONCLUSION

- Thanks the patient and explains that the examination is over
- Offers to help the patient to dress
- Washes hands

DISCUSSION

- Presents findings in a concise and confident manner
- Offers (differential) diagnosis

OVERALL IMPRESSION

- Treats the patient with dignity and respect at all times
- Demonstrates good communication skills
- Performs the examination in a fluent and professional manner

Thyroid Examination
Example Marking Scheme

BEFORE STARTING

- Washes hands
- Introduces self to the patient and states role
- Offers explanation and obtains consent
- Exposes the patient appropriately
- Positions the patient correctly (seated, with access to approach the patient from behind)
- Asks whether the patient is in any pain before examining

PERIPHERAL EXAMINATION

- Inspects the patient from the end of the bed for signs of thyroid disease, e.g. inappropriately dressed for climate; signs of anxiety or fidgeting; obvious swelling in the front of the neck
- Inspects nails for signs of thyroid acropachy
- Feels hands for temperature and clamminess
- Assesses the rate and rhythm of the radial pulse
- Examines for a postural tremor
- Inspects the face for signs of thyroid disease
  - ❱ looks for loss of the outer third of the eyebrows; facial puffiness or swelling; dry skin and hair
  - ❱ looks for exophthalmos, conjunctival oedema and lid retraction
  - ❱ tests for lid lag
  - ❱ examines eye movements for ophthalmoplegia
- Looks for pre-tibial myxoedema
- Tests for proximal myopathy
- States would elicit lower limb reflexes

EXAMINATION OF THE NECK
Inspection

- Inspects the neck
  - ❱ looks for scars, lumps or swellings
  - ❱ observes the neck while the patient swallows a sip of water
  - ❱ observes the neck while the patient protrudes their tongue

Palpation

- Asks whether there is any pain in the neck before starting
- Palpates any lump/swelling for consistency, size, tenderness and overlying skin temperature while positioned behind the patient
- Palpates lump/swelling as the patient swallows a sip of water
- Palpates lump/swelling as the patient protrudes their tongue
- Feels for submandibular and cervical lymphadenopathy
- Palpates the position of the trachea

Percussion

- Percusses over the lower neck and upper sternum

Auscultation

- Auscultates for thyroid bruits while the patient holds their breath in inspiration

ADDITIONAL POINTS

- States would perform Pemberton's test for superior vena caval obstruction
- States would like to perform thyroid function tests and an ultrasound examination of the gland with guided fine-needle aspiration cytology of any suspicious nodules

CONCLUSION

- Thanks the patient and explains that the examination is over
- Offers to help the patient to dress
- Washes hands

DISCUSSION

- Presents findings in a concise and confident manner
- Offers (differential) diagnosis

OVERALL IMPRESSION

- Treats the patient with dignity and respect at all times
- Demonstrates good communication skills
- Performs the examination in a fluent and professional manner

Peripheral Venous System Examination Example Marking Scheme

Remember that at every stage of the examination you should systematically compare one side with the other.

BEFORE STARTING

- Washes hands
- Introduces self to the patient and states role
- Offers explanation and obtains consent
- Exposes the patient appropriately
- Positions the patient correctly (standing initially, if possible)
- Asks whether the patient is in any pain before examining

INSPECTION

- Inspects the lower limbs
  - ❯ looks for peripheral oedema, bruising, varicosities, superficial thrombophlebitis, altered skin pigmentation, previous scars, venous eczema, ulcers, lipadermatosclerosis

PALPATION

- Asks whether the legs are painful before starting
- Feels the skin temperature of both lower limbs
- Palpates along the distributions of the short and long saphenous veins, observing the patient's face for signs of pain or discomfort
- Palpates over any varicosities for tenderness and temperature change
- Palpates for pitting oedema of the lower limbs bilaterally
- Locates the saphenofemoral junction (SFJ)
- Feels for a cough impulse at the SFJ

AUSCULTATION

- Auscultates for bruits over the SFJ

SPECIAL TESTS

- Performs tap test
- Performs tourniquet test (modified Trendelenburg's)
- States would perform modified Perthes test

ADDITIONAL POINTS

- States would like to examine the peripheral arterial system; perform an abdominal, pelvic and rectal examination, if indicated, to look for causes of inferior vena caval obstruction; and perform a Doppler ultrasound examination of the peripheral venous system

CONCLUSION

- Thanks the patient and explains that the examination is over
- Offers to help the patient to dress
- Washes hands

DISCUSSION

- Presents findings in a concise and confident manner
- Offers (differential) diagnosis

OVERALL IMPRESSION

- Treats the patient with dignity and respect at all times
- Demonstrates good communication skills
- Performs the examination in a fluent and professional manner

Peripheral Arterial System Examination Example Marking Scheme

Remember that at every stage of the examination you should systematically compare one side with the other.

BEFORE STARTING

- Washes hands
- Introduces self to the patient and states role
- Offers explanation and obtains consent
- Exposes the patient appropriately
- Positions the patient correctly (supine with one pillow)
- Asks whether the patient is in any pain before examining

INSPECTION

- Inspects surroundings for evidence to support a diagnosis of peripheral arterial disease, e.g. walking aids; cigarettes; blood glucose testing kit; glyceryl trinitrate spray
- Inspects the lower limbs
  - ❯ looks for amputations; previous scars; colour changes; loss of limb hair; skin texture and integrity; ulcers; gangrene

PALPATION

- Asks whether the legs are painful before starting
- Feels the skin temperature
- Measures capillary refill time of the toenails bilaterally
- Examines peripheral pulses
  - ❯ femoral
  - ❯ popliteal
  - ❯ posterior tibialis
  - ❯ dorsalis pedis
- Palpates abdominal aorta

AUSCULTATION

- Auscultates for abdominal aortic and femoral bruits

SPECIAL TESTS

- Performs Buerger's test
  - ❱ measures Buerger's angle
  - ❱ tests for reactive hyperaemia

ADDITIONAL POINTS

- States would like to examine the peripheral arterial system of the upper limbs and the cardiovascular system; perform a peripheral venous examination; and measure the ankle brachial pressure index (ABPI)

CONCLUSION

- Thanks the patient and explains that the examination is over
- Offers to help the patient to dress
- Washes hands

DISCUSSION

- Presents findings in a concise and confident manner
- Offers (differential) diagnosis

OVERALL IMPRESSION

- Treats the patient with dignity and respect at all times
- Demonstrates good communication skills
- Performs the examination in a fluent and professional manner

Inguinal Hernia Examination Example Marking Scheme

BEFORE STARTING

- Washes hands
- Introduces self to the patient and states role
- Offers explanation and obtains consent
- Exposes the patient appropriately
- Positions the patient correctly (standing initially, if possible)
- Asks whether the patient is in any pain before examining

INSPECTION

- Inspects the abdomen and both inguinal regions with the patient standing
  -) looks for previous scars and obvious swellings
  -) if swelling present, looks for erythema of the overlying skin
  -) observes the effects of coughing on the lower abdomen and inguinal areas, noting the direction of any protrusions

PALPATION

- Asks whether lower abdominal and inguinal areas are painful before starting
- Examines both inguinal regions with the patient initially standing and then lying
  -) feels for cough impulse over inguinal regions
  -) palpates any swellings for tenderness and difference in overlying skin temperature
  -) assesses reducibility of any swelling
    - — asks the patient to reduce the swelling themselves initially
    - — if the patient is unable to, offers to reduce the swelling
- Observes patient for any discomfort/pain during examination

PERCUSSION

- Percusses any swellings

AUSCULTATION

- Auscultates over any swellings

SPECIAL TESTS (*SEE* FIGURE 11)

- Attempts to differentiate between an inguinal hernia and a femoral hernia
  - ❭ locates pubic tubercle and asks the patient to cough, looking for the site of protrusion of the swelling in relation to pubic tubercle
- Attempts to differentiate between an indirect and direct inguinal hernia
  - ❭ reduces hernia and occludes deep inguinal ring (mid point of the inguinal ligament)
  - ❭ asks the patient to cough; if a cough impulse is palpable but the swelling does not reappear, then it is likely to be an indirect inguinal hernia

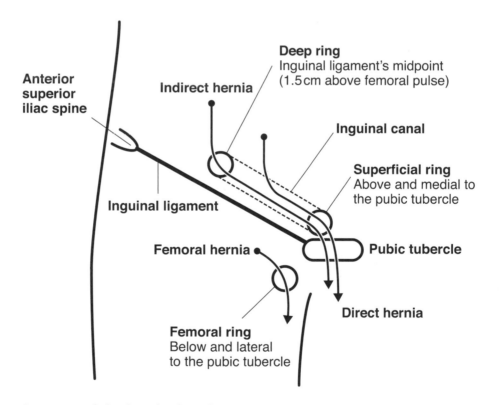

FIGURE 11 Anatomy of the inguinal region

ADDITIONAL POINTS

- States would like to examine the opposite inguinal region, abdomen and external genitalia

CONCLUSION

- Thanks the patient and explains that the examination is over
- Offers to help the patient to dress
- Washes hands

DISCUSSION

- Presents findings in a concise and confident manner
- Offers (differential) diagnosis

OVERALL IMPRESSION

- Treats the patient with dignity and respect at all times
- Demonstrates good communication skills
- Performs the examination in a fluent and professional manner

Case 43

Candidate instruction: Please examine this patient's abdomen

Patient information: Mrs H, a 42-year-old woman

Significant findings on examination:

Inspection:
Well-healed midline laparotomy scar
Stoma in RIF:
- stoma pink with no signs of necrosis
- spouted with single lumen
- semi-liquid stool in stoma bag

Peripheral examination: No abnormalities detected

Palpation: No abnormalities detected

Percussion: No abnormalities detected

Auscultation: No abnormalities detected

Important negative findings on examination:

No other abdominal scars
No erythema of the skin surrounding the stoma
No parastomal hernias
No abdominal discomfort/guarding on palpation
No abdominal masses or organomegaly
No ascites
Bowel sounds normal

Present your findings ...

Case 43 Diagnosis:

PREVIOUS LAPAROTOMY WITH END ILEOSTOMY

QUESTION 1

What are the likely conditions that may have resulted in this surgery?

QUESTION 2

How can you differentiate between an ileostomy and a colostomy?

QUESTION 3

What symptoms would indicate that a patient had a mechanical intestinal obstruction?

If there is a stoma present, check for the presence of a parastomal hernia

Case 44

Candidate instruction:	Please examine this patient's lower limb peripheral arterial system

Patient information: Mr O, a 68-year-old man

Significant findings on examination:

Inspection:	Tar staining of the fingers Shiny skin over the distal shins bilaterally

Palpation:	Temperature of right foot cooler than that of the left foot Temperature of both feet cooler than that of the shins Capillary refill time: • right foot, 4 seconds • left foot, 3 seconds

Pulses:	Left	Right
• Femoral	Palpable	Palpable
• Popliteal	Not palpable	Not palpable
• Posterior tibialis	Not palpable	Not palpable
• Dorsalis pedis	Not palpable	Not palpable

Auscultation:	No abnormalities detected

Special tests:	Buerger's angle: • 35° on the right leg • 45° on the left leg Buerger's test positive bilaterally

Important negative findings on examination:

No ulcers or gangrene
No signs of acute lower limb ischaemia
No abdominal aortic aneurysm palpable
No femoral bruits

Present your findings ...

Case 44 Diagnosis:

BILATERAL LOWER LIMB
PERIPHERAL ARTERIAL DISEASE

QUESTION 1

What simple bedside investigation could you do on this patient to assess the status of his lower limb peripheral arterial system?

QUESTION 2

What are the features of acute limb ischaemia?

The dorsalis pedis pulse is palpable just lateral to the extensor hallucis longus tendon; you can pinpoint this tendon by getting the patient to dorsiflex their big toe

Case 45

Candidate instruction: Please examine this patient's abdomen

Patient information: Mr V, a 72-year-old man

Significant findings on examination:

Inspection: Swelling in the right groin more prominent on coughing

Palpation: Smooth, non-tender swelling in right groin:
- palpable cough impulse
- coughing causes the swelling to protrude medial and superior to pubic tubercle
- swelling reducible
- once reduced, applying pressure over the mid point of the inguinal ligament prevents re-emergence of the swelling on coughing

Percussion: No abnormalities detected

Auscultation: No abnormalities detected

Important negative findings on examination:

No scars
No redness or increase in skin temperature over the swelling
No signs of hernial obstruction or strangulation
Bowel sounds normal
No abnormalities on examination of the left groin
If examined, no abnormalities of the external genitalia

Present your findings ...

Case 45 Diagnosis:

RIGHT-SIDED INDIRECT INGUINAL HERNIA

QUESTION 1

How would you manage this patient?

QUESTION 2

What clinical features of a hernia should cause concern?

QUESTION 3

How can direct and indirect inguinal hernias be distinguished anatomically?

If you find an inguinal swelling, make sure you examine the other side carefully, as there may be bilateral hernias with one side more obvious than the other

Case 46

Candidate instruction:	Please perform a peripheral venous examination of this patient's lower limbs
Patient information:	Mrs P, a 67-year-old woman

Significant findings on examination:

Inspection:	Dilated, tortuous veins on the medial aspect of the right thigh and calf
Palpation:	Cough impulse at the SFJ Palpation of the varicosity: • normal skin temperature • produces mild discomfort
Auscultation:	No abnormalities detected
Special tests:	Tap test positive Tourniquet test • refilling of the varicosity is controlled with tourniquet at the level of the SFJ

Important negative findings on examination:

No scars, ulcers, venous eczema or altered skin pigmentation
No pitting oedema
No signs of deep venous thrombosis
If performed, modified Perthes test negative

Present your findings ...

Case 46 Diagnosis:

VARICOSITY OF THE RIGHT LONG SAPHENOUS VEIN

QUESTION 1

How would you manage this patient?

QUESTION 2

What is the significance of Perthes test?

In patients with chronic venous disease, measuring the ABPI is helpful when assessing their suitability for compression bandaging or stockings

Case 47

Candidate instruction: Please examine this patient's abdomen

Patient information: Mrs B, a 70-year-old woman

Significant findings on examination:

Inspection: Well-healed midline laparotomy scar
Stoma in left iliac fossa:
- pink with no signs of necrosis
- non-spouted with a single lumen
- small amount of formed stool in stoma bag

Peripheral examination: No abnormalities detected

Palpation: No abnormalities detected

Percussion: No abnormalities detected

Auscultation: No abnormalities detected

Important negative findings on examination:

No other abdominal scars
No erythema of the skin surrounding the stoma
No parastomal hernias
No abdominal discomfort/guarding on palpation
No abdominal masses or organomegaly
No ascites
Bowel sounds normal

Present your findings ...

Case 47 Diagnosis:

PREVIOUS LAPAROTOMY WITH END COLOSTOMY

QUESTION 1

What type of surgery is this patient likely to have had?

QUESTION 2

What complications are associated with the presence of stomas?

If trying to distinguish between a Hartmann's procedure and an abdominoperineal resection, offer to examine the perineum; in an abdominoperineal resection, the anal sphincters and rectum are removed so there would not be a perforate anus

Case 48

Candidate instruction: Please examine this patient's abdomen

Patient information: Mr G, a 64-year-old man

Significant findings on examination:

Inspection: Patient appears underweight

Peripheral examination: Tar staining of the fingers

Palpation: Pulsatile and expansile mass above the umbilicus
Pulsation in time with the carotid pulse
Mass is approximately 4 cm in diameter

Percussion: No abnormalities detected

Auscultation: No abnormalities detected

Important negative findings on examination:

No abdominal scars
No abdominal discomfort/guarding on palpation
No other abdominal masses or organomegaly
No ascites
Bowel sounds normal; no bruits

Present your findings ...

Case 48 Diagnosis:

ABDOMINAL AORTIC ANEURYSM

QUESTION 1

How might you differentiate between a palpable aorta of normal calibre, e.g. in a thin patient, and an abdominal aortic aneurysm?

QUESTION 2

What are the risk factors for developing, an abdominal aortic aneurysm?

When palpating an expansile mass, your fingers move outwards as well as upwards with the pulse, whereas a pulsatile mass only moves your fingers upwards

Case 49

Candidate instruction:	Please examine this patient's neck
Patient information:	Mrs L, a 45-year-old woman

Significant findings on examination:

Inspection:
Swelling to the right of the midline:
- moves upwards on swallowing
- does not move on tongue protrusion

Palpation:
Right-sided swelling:
- measures 3 × 3 cm; 2 cm from the midline
- smooth, non-tender and firm
- moves upwards on swallowing
- does not move on tongue protrusion

Percussion:
No abnormalities detected in the upper thorax

Auscultation:
No abnormalities detected

Special tests:
No abnormalities detected

Important negative findings on examination:

No signs of airway obstruction
No scars
No erythema or difference in skin temperature over nodule
No peripheral signs of thyroid disease
No cervical lymphadenopathy
If performed, Pemberton's sign negative

Present your findings ...

Case 49 Diagnosis:

RIGHT-SIDED THYROID NODULE; PATIENT CLINICALLY EUTHYROID

QUESTION 1

What is the differential diagnosis in this patient?

QUESTION 2

How might you investigate this patient?

> The thyroid should be palpated from behind; if the patient is sitting with their chair against a wall, move them before you start so you can approach them from behind

Case 50

Candidate instruction: Please examine this patient's abdomen

Patient information: Mrs R, a 68-year-old woman

Significant findings on examination:

Inspection:
Overweight
Multiple abdominal striae
Hypertrophic midline abdominal scar 12 cm in length
Swelling protrudes along the length of the scar on coughing and when patient raises her head off the bed

Palpation:
Swelling has a palpable cough impulse and self-reduces

Percussion:
No abnormalities detected

Auscultation:
No abnormalities detected

Important negative findings on examination:

No other abdominal scars
No abdominal discomfort/guarding on palpation
No abdominal masses or organomegaly
No ascites
Bowel sounds normal

Present your findings ...

Case 50 Diagnosis:

INCISIONAL HERNIA ASSOCIATED WITH LAPAROTOMY SCAR

QUESTION 1

What is the main difference between a hypertrophic and a keloid scar?

QUESTION 2

What risk factors may predispose a patient to develop an incisional hernia?

Comment on a patient's nutritional status, if relevant; obesity is a major factor in the development of incisional hernias

5 Handy Hints for the Surgical Station

1. If you see a surgical scar but you are not sure what operation was performed, use common sense to make an educated guess based on your knowledge of the underlying anatomy.

2. When performing an abdominal inspection, ask the patient to raise their head off the bed. This may reveal a divarication of the rectus that you might otherwise miss.

3. Read the station instructions carefully, e.g. if you are asked to examine the patient's neck, start by doing just that. If the neck examination suggests a thyroid problem, and you have time, offer to do a more detailed examination looking for additional features of thyroid disease. If, however, you are asked to examine the patient's thyroid, then it would be appropriate to start with the peripheral examination first.

4. The discussion following the surgical examination may veer towards the anatomical – so it would be wise to revise the relevant anatomy in parallel with your surgical revision, as it might be a tad rusty …

5. If you notice that limbs or any bits of limbs are missing when doing a peripheral arterial examination, do feel free to mention this, as the examiner may have noticed too!

Surgical Model Answers

Cases 43–50

Case 43

ANSWER 1

A permanent ileostomy is usually created after a panproctocolectomy; the indications for this procedure include:

- Ulcerative colitis
  - ❯ failed medical treatment
  - ❯ toxic megacolon
  - ❯ development of colorectal cancer
  - ❯ prophylaxis against development of colonic malignancy in long-standing disease
- Hereditary conditions associated with an increased risk of bowel cancer, e.g. familial adenomatous polyposis
  - ❯ treatment for colorectal cancer in an affected person
  - ❯ prophylaxis against the development of colonic malignancy
- Crohn's disease.

The indications for creation of a temporary ileostomy include:

- Colorectal cancer
- Complicated diverticular disease
- During construction of an ileo-anal pouch.

ANSWER 2

Ileostomies are typically:

- Located in the right lower quadrant
- Spouted
- Produce liquid/semi-liquid stool.

Colostomies are typically:

- Located in the left lower quadrant
- Flush to the skin
- Produce formed stool.

ANSWER 3

Symptoms of bowel obstruction vary depending on the level of obstruction and on whether the obstruction is partial or complete but can include:

- Vomiting
- Colicky abdominal pain
- Bloating due to abdominal distension
- Constipation and failure to pass flatus
- High-pitched, tinkling bowel sound.

Case 44

ANSWER 1

Measurement of the ABPI will help in the diagnosis of lower limb arterial disease.

$$ABPI = \frac{\text{Highest ankle systolic pressure}}{\text{Highest brachial systolic pressure}}$$

ANSWER 2

The features of acute limb ischaemia are (the 'six Ps'):

- Pulseless
- Pallor
- Paralysis
- Paraesthesia
- Pain
- Perishingly cold.

Case 45

ANSWER 1

The available management options for inguinal hernias include:

- Lifestyle advice, e.g. weight loss, smoking cessation, avoiding heavy lifting
- Optimising control of any likely precipitating factors, e.g. constipation, chronic cough
- Scrotal supports and trusses (while awaiting/unfit for surgery)
- Surgical repair of the hernia.

ANSWER 2

The worrying features of a hernia would include:

- Incarceration (hernia irreducible)
- Incarceration with symptoms and signs of bowel obstruction
- Strangulation (irreducibility; erythema of the overlying skin and extreme tenderness on palpation) with or without evidence of bowel obstruction.

ANSWER 3

Inguinal hernias can be defined anatomically by their relationship to the inferior epigastric vessels; indirect hernias are lateral to the inferior epigastric vessels, whereas direct hernias are medial to these vessels.

Case 46

ANSWER 1

- The interventional management options for varicose veins include:
  - ❱ endothermal ablation using radiofrequency or laser
  - ❱ sclerotherapy
  - ❱ vein stripping surgery.
- The non-interventional management options include:
  - ❱ lifestyle advice, e.g. weight loss, smoking cessation
  - ❱ compression bandaging/stockings but only if unsuitable for interventional treatment.

See NICE guideline CG168 (2013)[8] for further information on management options.

ANSWER 2

Perthes test helps to determine whether the deep venous system is intact, but a duplex ultrasound scan would need to be done to confirm the findings.

---

8 NICE. Varicose veins in the legs: the diagnosis and management of varicose veins; NICE guideline 168. London: NICE; 2013. www.nice.org.uk/guidance/CG168

Case 47

ANSWER 1

The combination of a laparotomy scar with an end colostomy would most commonly indicate that the patient had undergone:

- Resection of the rectosigmoid colon and closure of the rectal stump (Hartmann's procedure)
- An abdominoperineal resection.

ANSWER 2

In some patients, the presence of a stoma requires considerable psychological adjustment and can result in the development of mental health issues.

Early complications of stomas include:

- Ischaemia
- Bleeding at the stoma site
- Stomal dysfunction, e.g. high output
- Stomal retraction
- Obstruction.

Late complications include:

- Stomal prolapse
- Stenosis
- Fistulae formation
- Parastomal hernias
- Chronic dermatitis
- Obstruction.

Case 48

ANSWER 1

A normal abdominal aorta may be palpable as a pulsatile mass but would not be expansile.

ANSWER 2

The risk factors for developing an abdominal aortic aneurysm include:

- Male sex
- Increased age
- Smoking
- Systemic hypertension
- Positive family history (first-degree relatives)
- Pre-existing peripheral vascular disease
- Presence of connective tissue disorders, e.g. Marfan's syndrome.

Case 49

ANSWER 1

The differential diagnosis for a solitary thyroid nodule includes:

- Adenoma
- Cyst
- The only palpable nodule of a multinodular goitre
- Malignancy.

ANSWER 2

The investigation of a thyroid nodule would include:

- Taking a full history and undertaking a detailed clinical examination
- Thyroid function tests; serum T_3, T_4, thyroid-stimulating hormone and antithyroid antibodies
- Ultrasound scanning
- Radionuclide scanning with technetium/iodine
- Fine-needle aspiration.

Case 50

ANSWER 1

The main difference between a hypertrophic and a keloid scar is that the former remains within the original scar boundaries whereas the latter extends beyond them.

ANSWER 2

The risk factors for developing an incisional hernia include:

- Raised intra-abdominal pressure due to:
  - chronic constipation
  - heavy lifting
  - chronic coughing
  - obesity
  - pregnancy
  - ascites.
- Poor abdominal musculature due to:
  - pregnancies, particularly multiple births
  - obesity
  - long-standing/recurrent ascites
  - peritoneal dialysis.
- Poor wound healing due to:
  - wound infection
  - increasing age
  - cigarette smoking
  - malnutrition
  - diabetes mellitus
  - chronic liver or renal disease.
- The operative procedure:
  - suture material, suture technique and incision type and length.

CPD with Radcliffe

You can now use a selection of our books to achieve CPD (Continuing Professional Development) points through directed reading.

We provide a free online form and downloadable certificate for your appraisal portfolio. Look for the CPD logo and register with us at: www.radcliffehealth.com/cpd

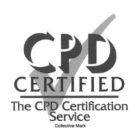